YOUR CAPILLARY QUOTIENT

The Hidden Secret in Cardiovascular Health

Carol Merlo, M.Ed., and Bill Merlo

Disclaimer

This book contains general information about medical conditions and possible treatments and does not constitute medical advice. Furthermore, you should only make medically based decisions based on the advice of your own trained physician. You should in no way delay or disregard seeking professional medical advice or discontinue it in any way once it has been given to you. In light of this clear medical disclaimer, the author and anyone or any entity related to them cannot be held legally accountable in any way for anything directly or indirectly related to the subjects discussed in this book.

Your Capillary Quotient: The Hidden Secret in Cardiovascular Health

ISBN: 978-1-7338553-2-7

Published by MPowered Press, Dallas, TX

TABLE OF CONTENTS

PREFACE

You certainly know how important cardiovascular health is. There is a good reason for that. According to the World Health Organization[1], cardiovascular diseases (CVDs) are the number one cause of death globally, taking an estimated 17.9 million lives each year.

Just about everyone has a parent or grandparent who has died from either a heart condition or a stroke. Carol was introduced to the effects of heart disease when she was a child. She remembers standing in a parking lot, looking up at the window of the hospital room where her grandfather was, after having had a heart attack. He was 63. At that time, no children were allowed in hospital rooms, so she didn't get to see him. A year or so after that, her great grandmother died of a stroke. This introduction made Carol acutely aware of the impact that cardiovascular health has on people.

As she grew, she learned more about her family's health. Her paternal grandfather dropped dead on the dance floor from a heart attack. He was in his fifties! Her mother, who had been devoted to diet and exercise, had a quadruple bypass in her seventies, which resulted in congestive heart failure. It deprived her brain of oxygen and caused her to have dementia. She progressively lost all her memories and died at 89 without being aware of any of her personal history.

Bill's father died in his sixties of a blood disorder but prior to that, he had had a heart attack. Bill's mother did, as well. His grandparents on both sides died of strokes.

These families are not unique. How many people do you know who are taking blood pressure medication and statins, or dealing with cardiovascular risk in some way?

Fortunately, modern allopathic medicine has done much to help people live with cardiovascular disease. Stents and bypasses are routinely administered to keep blood flowing. Medications can reduce clotting factors, reduce cholesterol, lower blood pressure, and improve blood flow. However, medications and surgeries aren't the best solutions because there are always risks and possible side effects to deal with, not to mention the costs involved.

Certain dietary supplements and alternative treatments have been shown to support and maintain the health of the cardiovascular system. This is often the way to go if you decide to be proactive and avoid the trip to the hospital and to an early grave. Even though modern medicine has so many treatments available, scientists agree that most cardiovascular diseases can be prevented by reducing behavioral risk factors such as tobacco use, unhealthy diet and obesity, physical inactivity, and the harmful use of alcohol.

Some of us do take care of ourselves but most of us don't. We have a serious obesity problem in the first world countries and most adults suffer from sedentary lifestyles. We sit in our cars, offices, and living rooms throughout the day and evening. The new catch phrase is that 'sitting is the new smoking[2].' More often than not, people rely on their doctors to handle the outcomes of this behavior.

Carol's first insight into this was when a close friend of hers had a heart attack. He was morbidly obese and had a heart attack in his late fifties. The doctors patched him up and sent him home with prescriptions for managing his heart and told him to diet and do exercise. He kept up with it for about four months and lost ten pounds. But then the old habits took over and so he continues to rely on medication, waiting for the next shoe to drop.

This disease is so insidious that we were confronted with it while writing this book. A routine checkup revealed that Bill's heart rate was slow, so he went to a cardiologist and discovered that he had an 80% blockage in one of his coronary arteries. As a result, he had to get a stent. Imagine if he had known about the Capillary

Quotient even a few years earlier! That is why we are passionate about getting younger people to check and track their microvascular health score.

WHY THIS BOOK?

There is an abundance of information out there on how to prevent cardiovascular disease. While valuable, this book introduces you to the importance of a little known or discussed part of the cardiovascular system: the microvascular (capillary) system. While medical doctors focus on the larger vessels and the heart, a more significant system may be failing you and doctors aren't treating it or are even aware of it!

One of the definitions of the word quotient is 'the magnitude of a specified characteristic or quality.' Think about an Intelligence Quotient (IQ). It is a measurement that indicates how well you can learn, understand, and apply information. Just like an IQ, the Capillary Quotient indicates how well your microvascular system works to maintain health.

By understanding the health of these microvessels, you can learn to live a longer, healthier life. Why? Because the microvascular system breaks down long before a doctor can detect any significant warning signs in your heart or larger vessels. When you are aware of this break down, you can take action before major damage occurs.

This book looks at the miraculous microvascular system and the communication that occurs in the body as a result of these capillary vessels. These vessels serve as the exchange portal that supplies nutrients and oxygen to the tissues while removing toxins and waste. The larger vessels and the heart pump are simply the gateway to and from the capillaries where the real work of supporting the health of the body is done.

We also want to arm you with ways you can test and improve your Capillary Quotient so that you can look and feel young, vibrant, and healthy throughout your life.

PART ONE: THE CARDIOVASCULAR SYSTEM

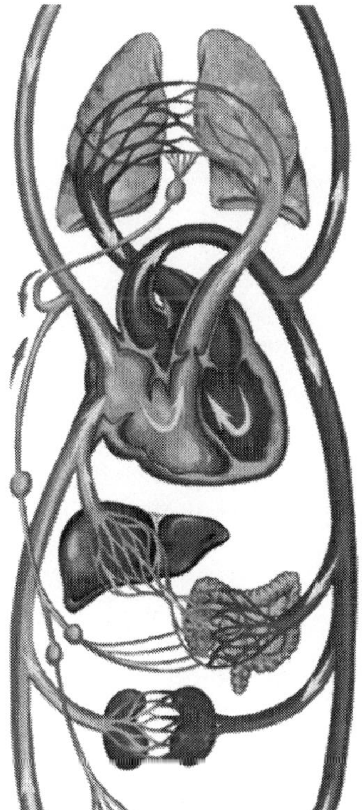

INTRODUCTION

Let's begin by looking at one of the most remarkable and efficient systems in the body, the cardiovascular system. The purpose of this system is to move blood. Blood flow determines the health and efficient functioning of every part of your body and is truly remarkable.

To give you an idea of how amazing it is, let's go on an imaginary trip from someone's work to their home. We first get on the freeway and drive for several miles at 75 mph. When we get to our exit, we'll take the off-ramp onto a side lane and slow down to maybe 45 mph. We then turn onto a 4-lane street for a little while at 40 mph and drive even more slowly onto our home street and enter the driveway. We are finally at home. Now, home is where the action happens. It's where we eat, drink, nourish ourselves, communicate with others, clean our bodies, eliminate our wastes, and throw out the trash. The drive home enabled us to get home and the beautiful system of roads got us there.

This is the perfect analogy for understanding our cardiovascular system. The large highways, feeder lanes. and streets are like the arteries, arterioles, veins, and venules of the MACROvascular system. These are primarily the blood's transportation network. And, like the neighborhood streets driveways and houses, the capillaries are the MICROvascular system where all the action happens. Here, the capillaries connect the blood flow to the cells (home), so that they can feed them with nutrients, oxygen, and hormones and cleansed by removing carbon dioxide, wastes, and toxins.

People know that they have capillaries but don't pay much attention to them. We think of the cardiovascular system as being composed of the heart and the blood vessels and don't really go beyond that., every one of these 49 hours are spent discussing the macrovascular system.

THE MACROVASCULAR SYSTEM

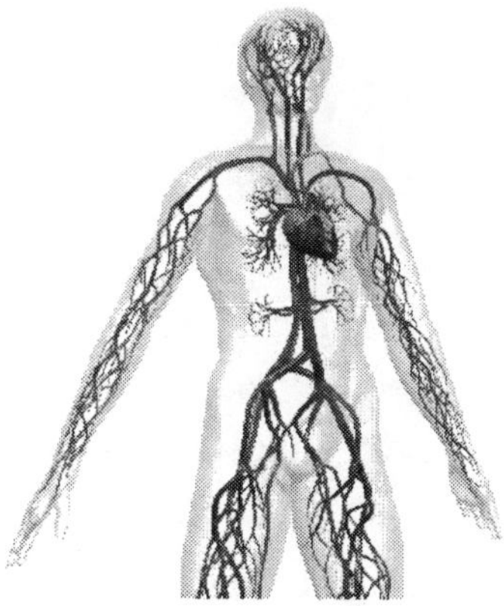

Your Amazing Heart

To think about your heart, just make a fist and look at it. Your fist is the size of your heart. The average adult heart beats around seventy times a minute, thirty-five million times a year, and two trillion times during an average lifespan[3]. It will pump 89 gallons of blood every hour and 2113 gallons of blood every day of your life. This amount of blood could fill one hundred swimming pools in a lifetime! It never loses its ability to pump blood throughout the body until the death of its owner.

The heart pumps by coordinating muscles on its right and left sides. On the heart's left side, the left atrium and ventricle distribute oxygenated blood to the organs and tissues. On the heart's right side, its right atrium and ventricle pump the oxygen-depleted blood to the lungs so it can be refreshed.

The heart is so intelligent it can figure out how much blood your body needs and pump just that much into your cells. The heart pumps between 1.057 to 1.585 gallons (4-6 liters) of blood a minute when you are at rest[4]. That is just enough because the resting body's cells don't require too much oxygen. If you are exercising, however, your need for oxygen rises. So, your heart beats faster and with the necessary force to meet the demand for energy. During exercise, the volume of blood pumped by your heart can increase by between four and seven times[4].

Heart Cells

These heart muscles are composed of cells that start beating about twenty-one days after conception. They can each beat on their own but sync up to work together. Heart muscle cells have a unique ability; they can shrink and expand. Even when you separate just one of those cells and place it under a microscope, it will continue to beat as long as you nourish it with blood[5]. Each cell in the heart produces the chemical energy that powers the heartbeat and keeps the life-giving blood assembly line moving throughout the body.

The Network that Feeds the Heart

The heart nourishes the body by pumping blood. However, it is an organ that also needs to be nourished. The heart requires enormous quantities of oxygen and nutrients to remain healthy. This is carried out through a special system that feeds it, called coronary circulation. As the blood leaves the heart to feed the rest of the body, it also moves through the coronary arteries to feed the heart muscle. The two coronary arteries, one for each side of the heart, receive oxygen-rich blood directly from the lungs and then return the blood directly to the lungs to be refreshed again, rather than going to through all the other organs. In this way, the blood richest in oxygen is continually devoted to nourishing the heart, itself.

Arteries

Blood leaves the heart through two arteries. The pulmonary artery sends the de-oxygenated blood from the heart to be revived in the lungs. The aorta is the largest artery and sends oxygenated blood from heart to the rest of the body. It holds a large amount of blood and is about an inch wide in a normal adult[7]. The aorta it is especially strong and elastic so that it can handle the pressure coming from the distribution of the blood from heart.

After the aorta leaves the heart, it divides into two branches of arteries: The upper branch goes to the head and arms, and the lower to various subsidiary vessels and organs.

Arteries have an elastic muscular structure that expands and to support the changes in blood pressure created by the heartbeats that move the blood through the system. Because of this, red blood cells can travel a long distance in a matter of seconds through the arteries.

Arterioles: Arterial Connection Points

The two branches of the arteries subdivide and thin out between six to eight times before they become arterioles. These are often referred to as feeder vessels, as they are found throughout the body and inside the organs that they supply with blood to feed the cells. Arterioles are the smallest branches in the arterial system—the arteries' final state before they branch into capillaries.

The arterioles have a powerful muscular system, like the arteries. They can close completely or widen, depending on demand of the local organ's need for oxygen and nutrients. This serves to attenuate the blood flow that reaches the capillaries so that the tissues receive only as much oxygen and nutrients as they need. This muscular system prevents the capillaries from being damaged by resisting the entry of high-pressure blood from the arteries. Each arteriole divides into branches that supply ten to one hundred capillaries, each.

The Venules and Veins: The Return Journey to the Heart

Once a red blood cell has delivered its oxygen, nutrients, and hormones, via the capillaries, it picks up carbon dioxide and other waste materials and starts its journey back through the venules to the veins. The carbon dioxide, wastes and toxins are then expelled through the lungs and kidneys, and the endless journey of the blood cells begins again. The red blood cells will perform this function as many as 1,000 times in a single day.

Instead of being red, the blood cells in your veins are purplish because they carry carbon dioxide instead of oxygen. The veins near your skin appear blue. In fact, the term 'blue bloods' originates from Spain to differentiate between the 'true' Castilians and those who intermarried with Moors, Jews, or other races. The expression probably originated in the visibility of the veins of people with lighter skin.

In terms of structure, the venules increasingly widen and become veins as the blood cells take their journey away from the capillaries back to the heart. Along the way, the veins widen to accommodate the number of blood cells coming into them. As venules become veins, they get progressively wider until they attach to the heart as two large veins. The maximum diameter in adults is a bit less than an inch, or 2.1 cm ± 0.7. One is called the superior vena cava (which means hollow vein). It comes from the head, arms, and upper body, and the other is called the inferior vena cava, which comes from the lower body.

The walls of veins are much thinner and less rigid than the walls of the arteries. The main reason for this is that the blood in the veins flows under much less pressure than in the arteries on its return journey. Its flow capacity is also aided by the action of one-way valves that restrict blood in the veins so that it can only flow toward the heart[6]. Because of these characteristics of less rigid, less pressure, and one-way valves, veins can hold almost seventy percent of the total blood volume of the body at any given time. This extra-venous volume is designed to have a reserve of blood available for emergencies and accidents.

Let's review some statistics, so you can gain an understanding of how utterly amazing this process is. The outflow and inflow of the blood is always balanced offset by volume and speed on each side.

- 84% of the entire blood in the body is in systemic circulation:
- 64% is on its journey back through the veins.
- 15% is moving through the arteries.
- 5% is moving through the capillaries.
- Of the remaining 16% of the blood supply:
- 7% is circulating in the heart.
- 9% is circulating in the pulmonary vessels (lungs).

THE MICROVASCULAR SYSTEM

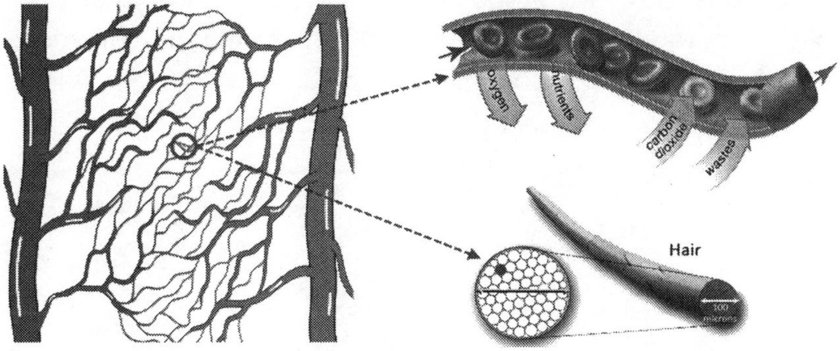

Each part of the cardiovascular system we've discussed so far is designed so that the capillaries can do their work. The microvascular system is composed of the capillaries. Capillaries are an intricate web of tiny vessels throughout your body that transport the blood from the arteries and facilitate the exchange of:

- nutrients,
- gases (such as oxygen and carbon dioxide),
- wastes (byproducts and toxins)
- other signaling molecules

and then return the blood back to the veins. It is the capillaries that function to supports the life of every cell, tissue, and organ in the body.

The Anatomy of the Capillary

Capillaries, like the other vessels, are tubes that the blood runs through.

- The inside space where the blood flows is called the lumen.

- The walls of these tubes are composed of individual endothelial cells that are collectively called the endothelium.
- The endothelium is the 'skin' of the capillary.

Since the purpose of the capillary is to allow components to be exchanged through the blood system, the endothelium has various gateway methods depending on what is being transferred and where they are being exchanged.

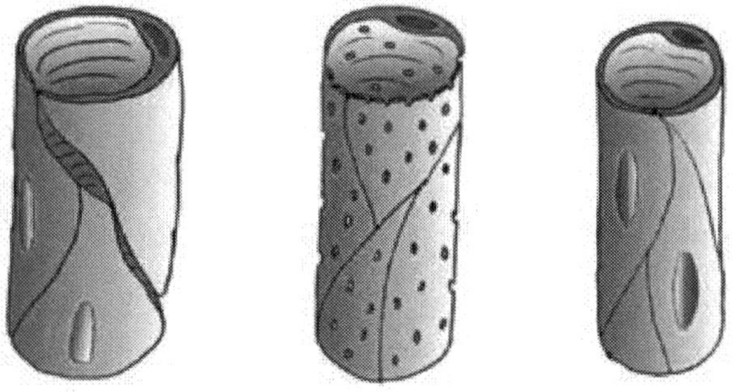

Various organs require different sized intercellular gaps between the neighboring endothelial cells. These gaps allow for the transport of fluids and larger molecules to and from blood and tissue. For example, the liver and spleen need large gaps, the kidneys and intestinal villi have smaller gaps and pores for filtration while muscle, nerve and brain have no gaps. These are referred to as 'tight junctions' and protect the blood-brain barrier.

In addition to the gaps, O2 and CO2 (gases), as well as other small lipid soluble substances permeate through the endothelium wall in a process called diffusion. The capillary structure also other pathways that enable the movement of even larger molecules through the capillary walls to deliver nutrients and hormones, and to remove toxins and waste from the surrounding cells.

Regardless of the method, the main function of capillaries is to move substances from one location to another.

Capillaries:

- ensure that fluids, oxygen, nutrients, hormones, and other substances, like organ and gland signaling molecules, are delivered to the surrounding cells and tissues.
- enable carbon dioxide, toxins, and wastes produced by your surrounding cells and tissues are delivered to areas in the body that can dispose of them.

Capillary Size

Capillaries are tiny. They are measured in microns. One micron equals 1/1,000 of a millimeter or 0.00004 inches. Capillaries are four to seven microns across. In comparison, a human hair is about 100 microns in diameter. You could fit up to 500, 4-micron capillaries a human hair. Now that's small! In fact, they are so small that individual red blood cells must squeeze through the smallest capillaries in single file by distorting their shape.

What they lack in size, they make up for in quantity. Ten billion (10,000,000,000) capillary vessels provide the infrastructure for the blood to feed and cleanse every cell in every tissue and organ in the body. Over 65,000 miles of vessels, equivalent to twice around the earth, fit into the adult human body and link every one of its 100 trillion cells[7]. If spread out, the capillaries would have a total surface area of over 10,000 sq. ft, which is three times the size of the average home.

About five percent of the total blood volume moves through the junction points between the arteries and the veins (systemic capillaries) at any given time.

Capillary Blood Flow

Blood flow is determined by a number of factors. One of which is perfusion. Perfusion is the term that refers to the flow of blood through the capillaries to feed tissues and organs. When the blood is moving through the capillaries, the capillaries are perfused.

Perfusion is important because it determines the health of the cells that surround the capillaries. This is influenced by: the amount of blood they have access to and the amount of time they have access to it. If the capillary is not perfused or if the blood moves through the capillary too quickly, there is not enough access to the blood to properly feed and cleanse the tissues, and so, organ failure may result over time.

For example, when we when we exert ourselves in any way beyond our relaxed state, such as during exercise, our heart responds by pumping blood more quickly through the body to supply our muscles and lungs with the nutrients and oxygen they need to handle the extra load.

In addition, blood flow is directed to the digestive tract after we eat. It flows to our extremities to warm us when we are cold and to our muscles when we exercise. When we are concentrating, the blood flow to the brain increases within a single second[9]. This extra blood flow is controlled and fed to the capillaries by the small arterioles to protect them from overload.

Healthy capillary beds have the ability to handle the extra flow needed to feed the tissues. First, each individual healthy capillary is covered with a thick, slippery, non-stick coating that enables increased blood flow to move through at higher speeds and volume. They also have something called a reserve capacity. This means that not all the capillaries are being used at full capacity at any one time. With exertion and more blood flow, more capillaries become perfused to handle the volume and ensure that red blood cells are traveling at proper speed.

Capillaries, Interstitial Fluid and Cells

If we consider that everything in the circulatory system begins and ends in the heart, then the capillaries are the midpoint of all this blood flow activity. Here, blood moves from the incoming arterial side to the outgoing venous side where the capillary enables the body's cells to be nourished, oxidized, and cleansed by the blood.

Capillaries do not need to touch every individual cell. Our 10 billion capillaries are so numerous that no cell in the body is more than 100 micrometers or 4/1000th of an inch away from a capillary. The exchange of materials between the capillary blood plasma and the nearby cells occurs through interstitial fluid, which surrounds nearly all the cells in the body. Interstitial fluid is the body fluid between blood vessels and cells, containing nutrients from capillaries by diffusion and holding waste products discharged out by cells due to metabolism. It consists primarily of water that dissolves nutrients, hormones, gases, wastes, and small proteins from the blood. The exchange of materials between capillary blood and nearby cells occurs through interstitial fluid which bathes nearly all the cells of the body.

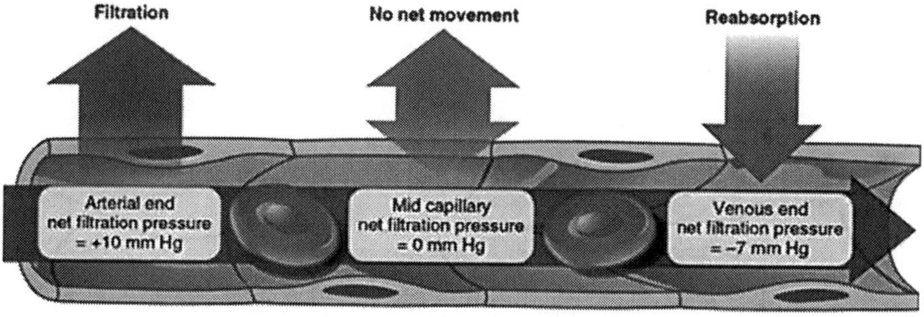

As you might recall, there are two systems of exchange: one for fluids and larger molecules moving through the intercellular gaps, and another for gases and small molecules that permeate directly through the endothelial cell membrane.

How is it that these constituents in capillaries can be moved into the cells and then back into these tiny micro vessels throughout the body?

For the fluids and larger molecules, the answer is in the pressures that are exerted inside and outside the capillary walls. On the outside of the capillary walls, the interstitial fluid applies constant pressure that pushes into the capillary wall. In contrast, on the inside, the blood pressure pushes out against capillary walls, but it is not constant. Since the entrance (arterial side) of the capillary is closer to the heart, the blood pressure is strong. It is greater than the outside pressure. This results in an outward flow of the nutrients from the capillary lumen to the interstitium called filtration.

At the midpoint of the capillary the pressures are balanced and there is no net movement, either in or out. Then, as the blood leaves the capillary (venous side) and moves toward the heart and into the larger returning blood supply, the blood pressure is less than outside pressure and the balance shifts to inward flow, drawing in wastes and other constituents from the interstitial fluid. This is called reabsorption. This balance between the capillary's internal pressure and interstitial external pressure maintains the outflows and inflows necessary to nourish and cleanse the cells.

Gases and smaller molecules, however, permeate through the endothelial cells because **molecules flow from a higher to a lower concentration**. Fresh blood in the arterial side of the capillary has a higher concentration of oxygen than that in the interstitial fluid. Consequently, oxygen will flow from the red blood cells out into the interstitial fluid to bathe the tissues, because interstitial fluid has a lower concentration of oxygen.

The cells in the interstitial fluid take in the oxygen, use it, and release carbon dioxide back into the interstitial fluid. The interstitial fluid now has a higher concentration of carbon dioxide than that in the red blood cells, so carbon dioxide flows back to the lower concentration in the red blood cells and back to the lungs to be reoxygenated and start this miraculous process all over again.

The Lymphatic System

While the capillaries remove waste and cleanse the cells, there is another contributing system that is equally important to your health. The lymphatic system has been referred to as the body's sewer system[8]. It maintains the proper fluid levels in our body by removing these excess fluids that leak out from our blood vessels. It also removes cellular wastes, absorbs digestive fats, is part of our immune system and protects our bodies from illness causing invaders.

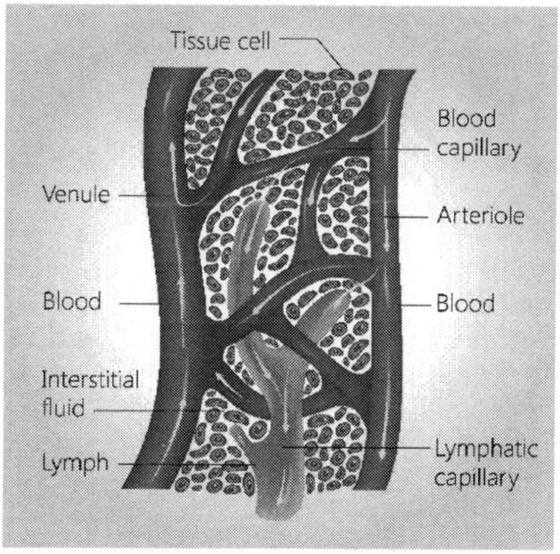

Similar to the pressure flows in the capillaries, the lymphatic system has an outward filtration pressure that is greater than the net inward reabsorption pressure. This causes a greater amount of fluid to be filtered out than that which is reabsorbed back into it. Any excess fluid that is not reabsorbed or used to feed tissue cells returns to the blood by way of the lymphatic system. The extra fluid that is left in the tissues accounts for approximately 15% of the capillary exchange.

The Body World Exhibition

The Body World Exhibition is a remarkable exhibit[9]. Here you can see cadavers in various states that underwent a process called plastination. After being plasticized, the bodies of some are cut into slices so that you can view the amazing biological processes that occur in the body.

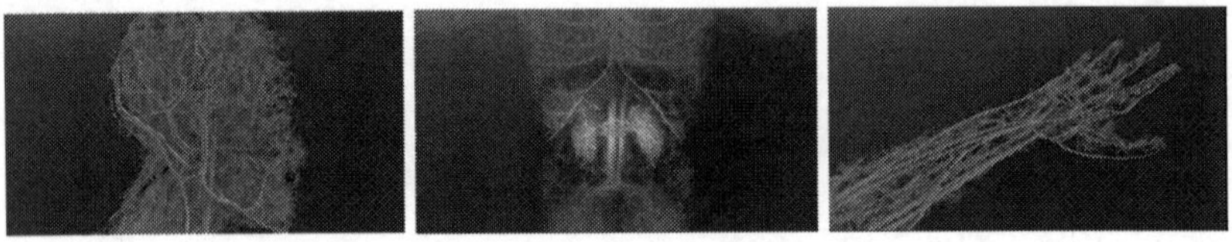

What you see in this image shows just the feeder vessels because the plastic could not fill the smallest, 4-to-9-micron level vessels. The vessels shown here are probably 10-12 microns across[10]. Regardless, you can clearly see the grouping of capillaries that feeds the organs. Every organ is filled with capillaries.

This very same phenomenon is happening in your own body! Consider how intricate and marvelous this micro vessel system is. We now understand the importance of these tiny vessels because of recent advancements in science and technology and recognize just how important they are to our overall health and longevity.

Capillaries Feed and Cleanse All Organs

A healthy blood flow through the capillaries ensures that cells are properly fed and cleansed to support healthy tissues, organs, and bodies. Unfortunately, this often does not occur. Damage or the shutdown of capillaries will lead to cell death, tissue and organ starvation, and disease. It is important to watch for signs like fatigue, cold hands and feet, or lack of focus so that you can avoid the bigger concerns like angina, heart attacks, or strokes. It is imperative that you support and keep your microvascular system healthy.

Capillary Facts

- It is estimated that the total length of capillaries in the human is over 65,000 miles.
- There are 300 million capillaries in the lungs, alone. If they were laid out, end to end, they would stretch 1,491 miles, roughly the distance between Los Angeles and Dallas.
- The capillaries in the brain are around 403 miles long. In contrast, the distance between Los Angeles and San Francisco is only 382 miles.

BLOOD: THE ELIXIR OF LIFE

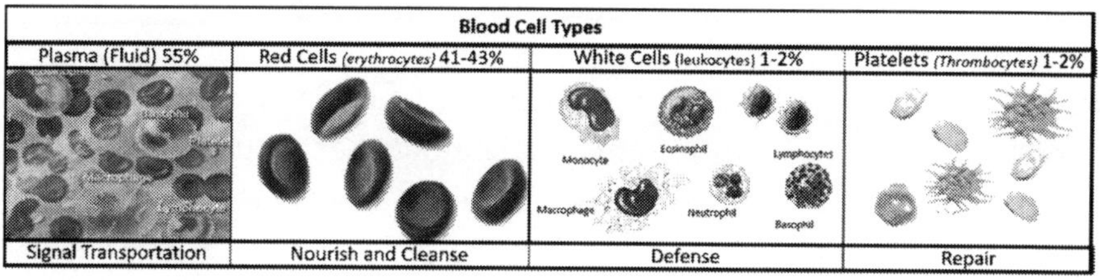

One key word keeps popping up in everything we've discussed so far: BLOOD. The term 'Life Blood' means just that; for surely, without blood there is no life. As we've mentioned, the heart and larger vessels are about transporting the blood to and from the capillaries. And, as you have learned, the capillaries are about the exchange that takes place between blood cells and tissues.

Because of this amazing microvascular infrastructure, blood—the liquid of life—can deliver oxygen and nutrients to all the cells in your body. The blood acts as both a carrier and a regulator in the body. It flows constantly, performing its tasks at every moment throughout that journey:

- Your blood is essential for nearly all the communication process inside the body.
- All the raw materials that the cells, and therefore for the body, needs are transported in the blood.
- The blood adjusts and maintains the body's temperature just like a thermostat.
- The defense antibodies and white cells in the blood are on constant duty, guarding against any invaders.
- The blood in your arteries supplies all the body's oxygen and nutrition.
- The blood in the veins acts as a sewage system that removes any waste products and toxins from the cells.
- The blood also has a mechanism for recognition, repair, and rejuvenation, in the vessels and surrounding tissue and organ cells.

Plasma: The Ocean of the Blood Stream

Each particle and cell in the blood is floating in a sea of plasma. The blood is composed primarily of red and white blood cells, stem cells, and hormone signaling molecules. In biology, cell signaling, or cell-cell communication, governs the basic activities of cells and coordinates multiple-cell actions. Signaling molecules interact with a target cell as a ligand to cell surface receptors, and/or by entering into the cell through its membrane. Blood also contains the platelets that clot the blood, proteins like albumin, fats like cholesterol, and debris composed of bacteria, viruses, parasites, dead cell components, and even fat particles.

Plasma constitutes 55% of the blood; 90% of it is water. The water in the plasma is the basic element of the blood. Since plasma is the fluid component of blood, its level can decline by up to 50% when you sweat, or it can rise by 60% when you hydrate. This is why hydration is so important--it keeps the blood fluid and moving.

Red Blood Cells (Nourish and Cleanse)

Red blood cells (erythrocytes) are the most numerous cells in the blood. Adult humans have about 20-30 trillion red blood cells at any given time, which is approximately one quarter of the total number of cells in the body. Red blood cells comprise approximately 90% of the cells in a drop of blood. Stretched end to end, these cells would form a tower 31,070 miles high. If we were able to spread them out like a carpet, they would cover 1,467 square miles[11].

Each red blood cell has a life span of around one hundred to one hundred twenty days. During its lifespan, a single red blood cell travels between the lungs and the other tissues of the body 75,000 times. By the time you read this page, you will have lost some three million red blood cells throughout your body. At the same time, a similar number will also have been produced in your bone marrow.

Red blood cells are produced by stem cells in the bone marrow. Although they *are* considered cells, red blood cells can't divide or replicate like other cells in the body. Mature red blood cells don't have nuclei. When they enter the bloodstream for the first time, they eject their nuclei and organelles, so they can carry more *hemoglobin,* and thus, more oxygen[12].

Why Are Red Blood Cells Flat Instead of Spheric?

Red blood cells are shaped like a disc. This allows red blood cells to open a wide space inside themselves to make room for the nearly 300 million hemoglobin molecules that get packed into any single red blood cell. These hemoglobin molecules can take up 90% of the space in a single red blood cell[13].

Many factors enable red blood cells to carry oxygen, and all of them are essential. One is their flattened shape. This shape increases the cell's surface area and facilitates contact with oxygen molecules, as well as making it easy for the cell to deposit oxygen at the right time and in the right place. Thanks to its shape, the red blood cell can load up with far more oxygen molecules than it could if it were shaped like an ordinary eukaryotic cell. Eukaryotic cells are round and contain a nucleus, as well as organelles, and look like the cells you see in a biology textbook.

Some capillaries are only 4-5 microns (micrometers) wide, which is too narrow for red blood cells with a diameter of 7 to 8 microns. Because of their unique shape, red blood cells can compress themselves to enter small spaces. Since they have a large cell membrane in proportion to the amount of volume they carry, red blood cells can easily change their shape to reach these small areas of the body.

Hemoglobin

Hemoglobin gives your blood its red color. Its function is to keep every cell in your body alive. It transports oxygen to the cells and picks up the carbon dioxide that the cells need to discard. Hemoglobin is an extraordinary molecule because it can perform different jobs at the same time. First, it can select out oxygen from the millions of molecules passing through the capillary vessels in the lungs. Hemoglobin has an amazing oxygen-carrying ability, which enables it to bind four separate oxygen molecules. These oxygen molecules are released through the microvascular circulation to support various organs and tissue cells where they are needed and when they are needed.

Second, hemoglobin collects the carbon dioxide molecules from the cells. Carbon dioxide also attaches to hemoglobin from the tissues with a rather weak bond, so that it can be returned to and refreshed by the lungs. Red blood cells can carry much larger quantities of carbon dioxide than they can of oxygen.

What Happens to Red Blood Cells at the End of Their Life Span?

Red blood cells that have come to the end of their lives are broken down by the large white macrophage blood cells in the liver, spleen, and bone marrow, where the hemoglobin in the dead red blood cell is released. Over the ensuing few hours, the macrophages separate the iron from the hemoglobin to be carried in the bloodstream—either to the bone marrow to produce new red blood cells, or to the iron storage areas in the liver and other tissues for use at a later date. The macrophages convert the rest of the hemoglobin molecule into a bile pigment to be excreted.

White Blood Cells (Defense)

White blood cells (leukocytes) are the body's armed forces. Potential invaders are everywhere and pose a threat to your health when they are ingested. Do you realize how many foreign substances there can be in a delicious meal you eat, the air you breathe, the water your drink, or the people you shake hands with?

The white blood cells identify and eliminate toxins. These amazing cells wage war on all kinds of foreign bodies. Like the army, there are several divisions of white cells: each with a different target and purpose. Some fight germs directly, while others patrol the body and recognize foreign molecules and microbes that need to be destroyed.

White blood cells are produced in the bone marrow at a production rate of 1.2 million a second. The bone marrow stores an estimated 80–90% of white blood cells it has made. When an infection or inflammatory condition is spotted by the protector cells, the body releases the defenders into the bloodstream, where they can kill 'the enemy.'

The other 10-20 percent of the leukocytes circulate in the blood plasma, standing by to be ready to attack as soon as they are needed. The white cells' journey to and from the heart to the head is around ten seconds. It takes roughly one minute for it to arrive at the big toe.

Once they enter the bloodstream from the bone marrow, the leukocytes' lifespan is from three to four hours in blood and three to four days in tissues. If there is a severe infection, the leukocytes will only live for an hour or two. That is because they travel toward those areas of the body that are under attack, defend the body, and then either die of exhaustion or of poisoning by the invader. If there is no infection or invader, the protector cells visit every one of the 100 trillion cells in the body several times a day—during which they identify and eliminate sick or aged cells. The defender cells attack, engulf, or eat the invaders or the diseased cells. The protector cells send signaling molecules to the defender cells when they find the enemy.

There are several types of white blood cells:

- **Leukocytes**, a white (blood) cell; are a colorless cell that circulates in the blood and body fluids and is involved in counteracting foreign substances and disease. There are several types, including lymphocytes, granulocytes, monocytes, and macrophages.
- **Neutrophils** (Defender Cells) are the most common, comprising about 50-60% of all the circulating leukocytes. They are the first line of defense, which work against infectious agents or other 'non-self' substances and are about twice the size of red blood cells. They are attracted by the chemicals released by bacteria which draws them to an infection to engulf and destroy it in a process called phagocytosis.
- **Lymphocytes** (Protector Cells) are the second most common. Lymphocytes produce antibodies, which fight against infections from viruses.
- **Monocytes** (Trash Collectors) are the third type. They can form into macrophages, which are large white cells. Macrophage means 'Big Eater'. They identify, attack, and engulf bacteria, viruses, pieces of old cells, and other invaders, consuming them. Since macrophages are larger than neutrophils, they can consume a greater number of invader pathogens.

As opposed to the red blood cells, white blood cells are eukaryotic cells because they contain a nucleus. Under normal conditions, a pint of blood contains between 3,000 and 5,000 white blood cells and 2.4 trillion red blood cells. That's an average of 500 red blood cells for every white one. If all the leukocytes (white blood cells) in the bloodstream were to be gathered, they would just about fill a coffee cup.

Platelets (Repair)

Platelets (thrombocytes) are another essential element in the blood. Platelets are small disks that break off from large cells in the bone marrow. One drop of plasma contains more than one hundred million platelets. These are small, colorless cell fragments in our blood that form clots to stop or prevent bleeding. If you start to bleed, the damaged area sends out signals to the platelets. The platelets then rush to the wound and begin to stick to one another as well as to the blood vessel wall. At the same time, a chemical in the plasma changes and hardens into thin threads called fibrin. These threads trap the platelets and blood cells to form a clot. The clot seals the leak and prevents further bleeding. Platelets live in the blood for seven to nine days.

Stem Cells (Build)

Stem cells are cells that can differentiate into several types of cells and reproduce indefinitely to make more of the same stem cell. Only one out of every 10,000 cells produced in the bone marrow is a stem cell—a ratio that sometimes falls to as low as one in 100,000. A stem cell determines the requirements inside the body and then either forms into the cells which replenish blood and immune cells or those that maintain bone, cartilage, muscle, and fat cells. The communication via signaling molecules that takes place in the blood determines when and how a stem cell will differentiate.

There is increasing evidence that the aging process can have adverse effects on stem cells. As stem cells age, their ability to renew deteriorates and their ability to differentiate into the various cell types alters. This is why people are now using injected or infused stem cells as medical treatments for repair and regeneration. They have been shown to help with a range of conditions including cancer and arthritis. You can choose to receive an injection of stem cells either into a specific area or as an infusion, which works more systemically.

Albumin (Transport)

Albumin has a particularly significant role in your health. It is the most abundant protein in plasma and transports cholesterol and hormones. In addition, it binds mercury and antibiotics. It releases toxins to the liver and carries nutrients, fats, and hormones to their requisite destinations.

Albumin plays an important role as a carrier protein for hormones, which impact your emotional health and energy levels. Hormones are responsible for the distribution of messages in the body and carry the vital messenger molecules in the albumin. They are responsible for signaling hunger and thirst, among other things. Without albumin, you wouldn't know when you were thirsty or hungry.

Albumin is also the main protein in plasma. It controls the outside-in pressure on the capillary from the interstitial fluid which draws water into the blood vessels. This process prevents excessive fluid leakage around the cells.

Now let's see how the capillaries use all of these blood constituents to manage our health by keeping our cells, tissues, and organs healthy.

SIGNALING MOLECULES IN CELLULAR COMMUNICATION

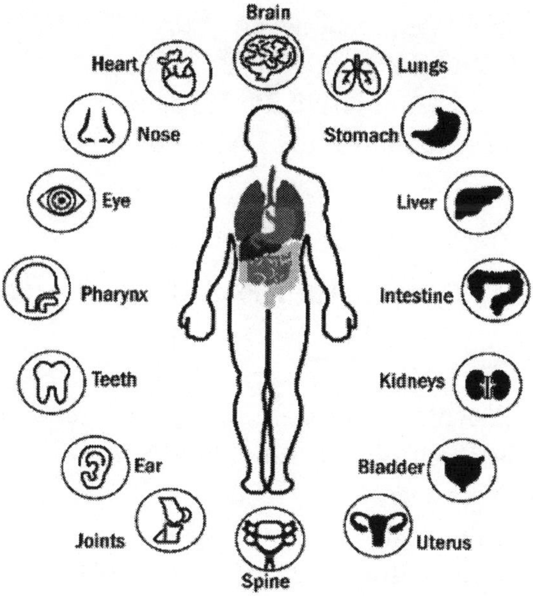

Throughout our conversation so far, we have described the microvascular system as a capillary exchange network. This amazing network feeds the cells by delivering oxygen and nutrients and cleanses them by removing carbon dioxide and wastes. Certainly, the process of the red and white blood cells, platelets, and plasma interacting with the body's cells is part of this communication network.

One aspect of cellular communication we have not touched on is the role of signaling molecules and how capillary health impacts their ability to do their job. Signaling molecules, generated by glands, fat, and bones are responsible for transmitting information between cells in your body. The size, shape, and function of different types of signaling molecules can vary greatly. All glands, organs, and cells communicate using these signaling molecules.

There are four major types of signaling mechanisms that occur in multicellular organisms. Each of these types facilitates the complex communications required to operate and control the body's functions:

1. paracrine (for example, between neurons),
2. endocrine (coming from glands),
3. autocrine (source and target are the same),
4. direct signaling (between the plasma membranes of neighboring cells).

How Signaling Molecules Work in Glands and Organs

A signaling molecule (technically called a ligand) is basically a messenger. It is produced, secreted, and sent to a target receptor which then triggers a series of reactions in the target cell, organ, or system. The beauty of this process is that the receptors are perfectly matched with the signaling molecules. This 'lock and key' structure on the surface of the cells enables the target receptor to identify and receive the messages from the signaling molecule.

How do these signaling molecules get to the right targets? They travel through the interstitial fluid, the rich network of the capillaries, and the vascular blood stream to find specific receptor cells located anywhere in the body. These signaling molecules are extremely small—about 100,000 times smaller than a grain of sand.

While this book cannot contain the information on every single function of the capillaries and signaling molecules, we are touching on those that are fascinating to us, and we hope they will be to you, too.

Endocrine System Signaling Molecules

Remember (yes, we know we sound like we are beating a drum, here) that systems, organs, and glands cannot be healthy unless they contain healthy capillaries. Glands are not like organs; they always secrete substances and send out signaling molecules. Like any other cell or tissue in the body, our glands are fed by nutrients and oxygen-rich blood. However, if the capillaries in the glands break down and get leaky, they will begin to starve and will no longer be able to deliver their hormones through the bloodstream[14]. This leads to the early warning signs like headaches, vision problems, high sugar levels, unexplained weight gain, loss of libido, feeling dizzy and nauseous, muscle wasting, and other not-so-fun experiences.

Signaling molecules from the glands do not just 'happen' to get into the bloodstream. They are delivered to the bloodstream through minute capillaries inside each gland. They travel through the other parts of the bloodstream until they reach an appropriate receptor cell, where they can perform the function dictated by the signaling molecules.

Here are some important endocrine glands and their signaling molecules:

The Pituitary Gland

This gland is located at the base of the brain, is often referred to as the most important part of the endocrine system. It produces hormones that control many of the functions of other endocrine glands by releasing a 'stimulating hormone' into circulation. This hormone signals the target gland to secrete its hormone[31].

THE THYROID GLAND

Another important endocrine gland is the thyroid. It secretes a signaling hormone called thyroxin. Thyroxin helps maintain blood pressure, heart rate, digestion, muscle tone, and reproductive functions. It also plays a role in bone growth and development of the brain and nervous system in children.

THE ADRENAL GLANDS

The adrenals are located on the top of the kidneys. You can think of them as 'Add Renal.' (Renal refers to the kidneys). These glands have a two-part function. The outer part (cortex) distributes corticosteroids, which are the signaling molecules that regulate the body's metabolism, balance of salt and water, immune system, and sexual function. The inner part (medulla) produces and distributes adrenaline, which help the body cope with physical and emotional stress by regulating heart rate, breathing rate, blood pressure, and carbohydrate metabolism.

THE PANCREAS

This gland is just below the stomach. It secretes insulin and glucagon into tiny capillaries buried in its islet cells. These hormones regulate the levels of glucose (sugar) in the blood. Type 1 Diabetes results from an increased plasma glucose concentration. Here, impaired capillaries lead to a deficiency in the production of insulin.

Organ System Signaling Molecules

The Gut – The Small Intestine Walls

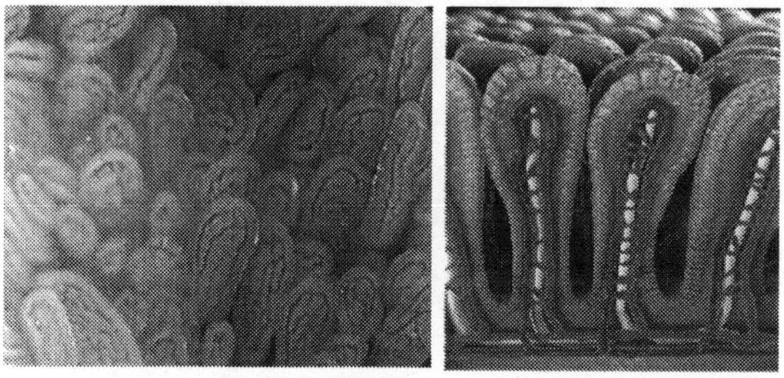

Everyone knows that we eat food that goes into our stomachs to get digested and then moves through our small intestines, which absorbs the nutrients. But how many people think about how those nutrients get absorbed and distributed to the rest of our body? The gut has capillaries that absorb the nutrition to pass on to the bloodstream, which feeds the body.

The average small intestine is twenty-two ft. in length with a surface area of 2,700 sq. ft. The inner lining of the small intestine is covered with a carpet of tiny projections called villi. The absorbed nutrients enter the bloodstream through these capillary beds inside each villus. As you can see in the above illustration, when nutrients are absorbed into a microvillus, they enter its capillary. This is how nutrients from your food enter your blood. By the time food leaves a healthy small intestine, all the nutrients in the food will have entered the bloodstream and been sent to the liver for processing.

These villi are necessary for digestion to occur. In people with gluten intolerance, the villi are completely flat and cannot easily absorb nutrients. 'Leaky gut,' is a condition where the carpet of villi has partially broken down so, there are holes in it where the villi would ordinarily be tightly packed. The more villi that break down, the fewer capillaries exist to absorb nutrients into the blood stream.

The villi also enable signaling molecules to pass from the gut into the blood stream. One example of this is the gut signaling molecule called leptin. After you have eaten, the intestinal cells burst out clouds of signaling molecules to the brain saying, "I am full."

Receptor cells in other organs respond to this message by controlling appetite or promoting nutrient absorption[15].

THE LIVER

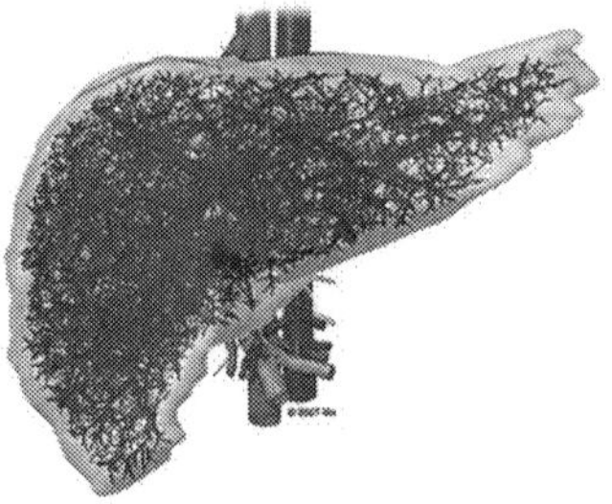

The capillaries in the liver receive the absorbed nutrients from the capillary beds in the gut villi. This capillary blood exchange in the liver metabolizes, or breaks down, nutrients from food to produce energy when it is needed and prevents shortages of nutrients by storing some vitamins, minerals, fats, and sugars. The liver also produces most of the substances that regulate blood clotting as well as bile, which is the compound needed to digest fat and to absorb vitamins A, D, E and K.

THE KIDNEYS

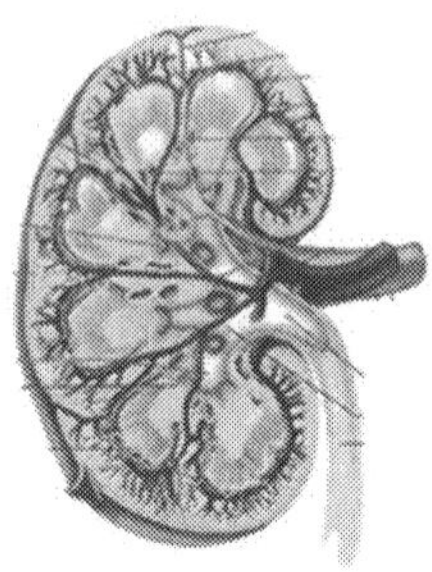

The capillaries keep the kidney tissue healthy. The body's capillaries collect carbon dioxide, toxins, and waste products from all the cells in the body and then deliver them via the blood stream to either the lungs for reoxygenation or to the kidneys and bladder, where they are eliminated. The kidneys are not just filters. The kidney capillaries also reabsorb useful substances, such as glucose and amino acids and other chemicals that keep the body in balance.

The kidneys hold a commanding position in the body's network of blood vessels. In fact, about one quarter (1/4) of the blood pumped by the heart goes to the kidneys because the fundamental job of the kidneys is the to manage the blood. The kidneys monitor the amounts of red blood cells in your body, manage your blood pressure, and send commands across the body.

Blood vessels function as the body's transportation routes and are also used as information circuits that carry signaling molecules. When the body is suffering oxygen deprivation, the kidneys start releasing a tiny signaling molecule which sends a message from the kidney capillaries to other organs, saying, "We need more oxygen." This message is picked up by the target receptor cells in the bones, which have holes in them that contain capillaries connected to the bone marrow, where blood is produced. The signaling molecule from the kidneys flows into the spaces within the bone and the message is picked up[32]. In response, red blood cells, the transporters of oxygen, start multiplying. This increase in the number of red blood cells enables more oxygen to be delivered to the muscles to answer the signaling molecule's request. Proper functioning kidneys with healthy capillaries are constantly sending out signals to our bones to keep our blood oxygen levels at an optimum.

Blood Chemical Levels

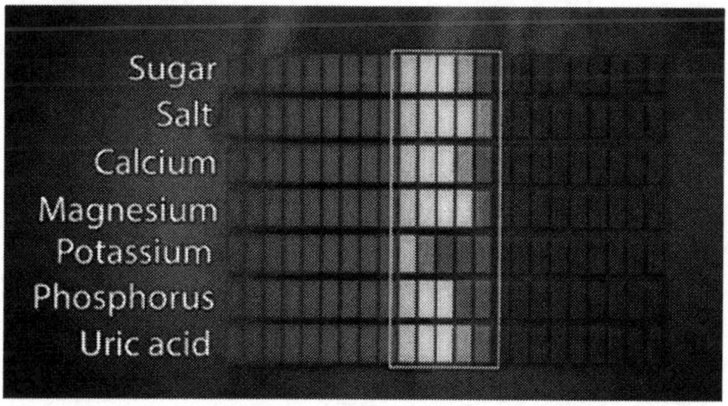

Our kidneys are also responsible for regulating blood chemical levels. They work constantly to fine tune the many types of chemicals in our blood. Each kidney contains about one million tightly-wound bundles of small capillary blood vessels called the glomerulus. These have been said to be the most intricate structure of any organ in the human body. Blood pressure pushes the water and solutes in the blood through these tiny capillary membranes that retain the desired essential chemicals and remove the waste as urine. Each day approximately fifty gallons of blood (180 liters) is filtered through these glomeruli capillaries, and yet, we only produce about one gallon (4 liters) of urine. The rest of the filtered and cleansed chemicals, such as sugar, salt, calcium, magnesium, potassium, phosphorus, and uric acid are reabsorbed, becoming fresh blood.

The kidneys and the kidney signaling molecules are key areas for overall wellness and longevity. By maintaining a proper blood flow through the healthy glycocalyx, capillaries regulate the components of our blood through this remarkable organ.

Bone Marrow

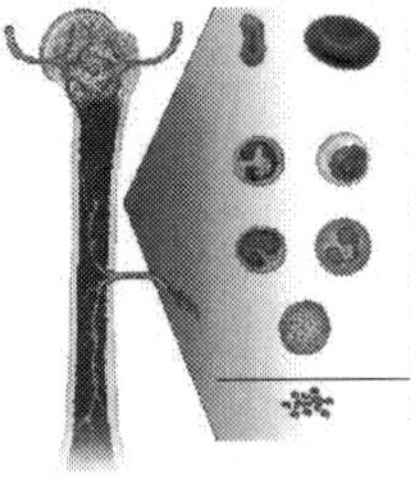

In the kidney section above, we discovered how a signaling molecule is sent from the kidney into a capillary, through the blood system and received by the bone marrow to help regulate the production of more red blood. Let's expand on that and dive in deeper to find out how bone signaling molecules can affect not only bone strength but also memory and longevity.

Bone marrow is the soft, spongy tissue inside your bones that makes new blood-forming stem cells. Remember that these cells transform into whatever type of blood cell is needed by the body and go exactly where needed to replace damaged or dead cells. The communication system dictates what cells to produce and delivers them where they are needed.

While bone marrow is not considered to be an organ, its microvasculature is significant and impacts overall health. The capillaries in your bones carry between 260 and 400 billion new blood cells into your blood stream each and every day.

If you look inside the bones, you will see big columns made up of calcium interlaced with strands of blood vessels and gelatinous marrow. There are also cells called osteoclasts that roam over the bone surface to break it down and dissolve the calcific surface. The bone then gets rebuilt by other cells called osteoblasts. They cram into cavities created by the osteoclasts and release a viscous liquid that hardens to form fresh bone tissue. This process of erosion and rebuilding keeps the bone strong and replaces your entire skeleton every five years.

In addition to building bones, osteoblasts send a signaling molecule that plays a critical role in directing memory, called osteocalcin. This ligand signaling molecule is released while the osteoblast is forming new bone. It moves through the interstitial fluid into the capillaries[16]. It is then carried through the bloodstream to the brain, where the message is delivered. Osteocalcin has a receptor in a part of the brain responsible for memory called the hippocampus, where the signaling molecule is released as part of the capillary exchange in the brain. The message boosts memory power.

The Antiaging Signaling Molecule

The messaging power in our bones isn't just limited to memory. The bones also release a signaling molecule called osteopontin. This molecule contains the messages connected to the process of aging. The message from osteopontin essentially boosts immunity. It gives rise to various immune cells, and the more immune cells that are created, the better our immune system functions. In addition, the messages from our bones can affect the testes in men to improve reproductive capabilities. They even work in our muscles to help increase stamina. These are all crucial factors in keeping us young. Scientists are now beginning to think that signaling molecules from our bones are responsible for our body's youthfulness!

The Lungs

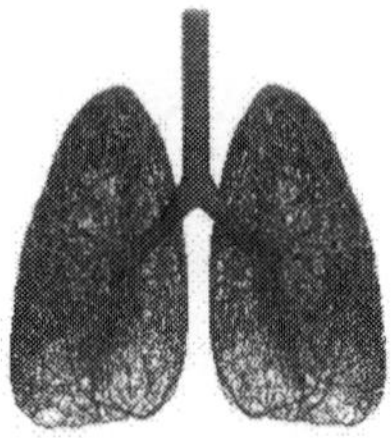

The lungs, alone, have over 300 million capillaries in them. If they were laid out end to end, they would stretch for 1,500 miles, the distance from San Diego to Seattle. Carbon dioxide is eliminated through the tiny capillaries in the walls of small sacs called alveoli, where the exchange with oxygen takes place. Cells can't live without the oxygen that is delivered through these capillaries.

The Brain

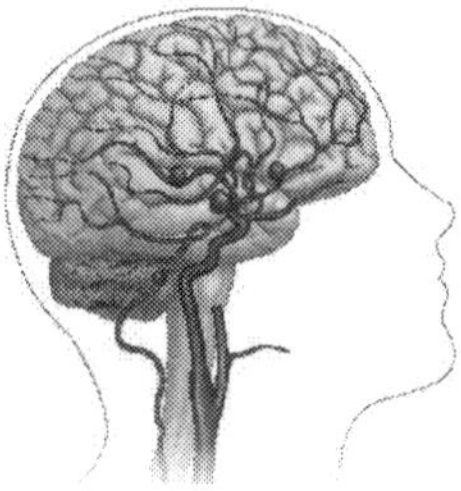

Your brain is an amazing organ that needs to be constantly fed and protected. It only takes up only two percent of the weight of an average adult, but it uses 20% of the body's energy and 20% of its oxygen. For this reason, the brain tissue receives 15 - 20% of the total cardiac output. The brain generates a tremendous amount of heat and metabolic waste. The capillaries in the brain deliver vital oxygen which enables you to think clearly. They form the blood–brain barrier. Here, the endothelial cells are wedged closely to each other, forming what are called tight junctions. These tight gaps only allow small molecules, fat-soluble molecules, and some gases (think oxygen and carbon dioxide) to pass freely through the capillary wall and into the brain tissue. Toxins and pathogens cannot pass through.

The brain manufactures signaling molecules called neurotransmitters. These are hormones that transmit signals from one neuron (brain cell) to another neuron, muscle cell, or gland cell. You have probably heard of some of them. For example, serotonin affects mood, appetite, and sleep, norepinephrine affects stress and blood pressure, dopamine is involved in cognition, motor control, motivation, and reward mechanisms, glutamate is involved in memory, and endorphins control your response to pain. Further, neurotransmitters in the peripheral and neural tissues support communication and coordination between several types of cells. They play a key role in inflammation, insulin sensitivity, and fat and energy metabolism.

As you can see, the health of your capillaries impacts each and every function of your body through signaling molecules. As we move into the next section, we will look at the structure and function of the capillaries and how that impacts your health.

REFERENCES PART ONE

1. Cardiovascular Diseases. (2017). World Health Organization. "https://www.who.int/en/news-room/fact-sheets/detail/cardiovascular-diseases-(cvds)
2. Baddeley, B., Sornalingam, S., & Cooper, M. (2016). Sitting is the new smoking: where do we stand? The British Journal of General Practice: The Journal of the Royal College of General Practitioners, 66(646), 258. https://doi.org/10.3399/bjgp16X685009
3. Simon, S. (1996). The Heart – Our Circulatory System. New York: Mulberry Books.
4. Guyton, A., and Hall J. (2001). Textbook of Medical Physiology. Saunders.
5. Poole, R., Editor. (1986) The Incredible Machine. National Geographic Society.
6. National Cancer Institute, Seer Training Modules. Classification & Structure of Blood Vessels. https://training.seer.cancer.gov/anatomy/cardiovascular/blood/classification.html
7. Beckerman, James Medical Reviewer. (2020). How the Heart Works. WebMD. https://www.webmd.com/heart-disease/guide/how-heart-works#1
8. The Great Lymphatic System, the Body's Sewer System. March 18, 2019. https://martinswellness.com/wellness-connection/lymphatic-system.html/
9. https://bodyworlds.com/.
10. ER Services. Anatomy and Physiology Module 4. The Cardiovascular System: Blood Vessels and Circulation. Capillary Exchange https://courses.lumenlearning.com/suny-ap2/chapter/capillary-exchange/#:~:text=Filtration%2C%20the%20movement%20of%20fluid,is%20driven%20by%20the%20BCOP.

11. Simon, S. (1996). The Heart – Our Circulatory System. New York: Mulberry Books.
12. LibreTexts. (2020).16.2A: RBC Anatomy. https://med.libretexts.org/Bookshelves/Anatomy_and_Physiology/Book%3A_Anatomy_and_Physiology_(Boundless)/16%3A_Cardiovascular_System_-_Blood/16.2%3A_Red_Blood_Cells/16.2A%3A_RBC_Anatomy.
13. University of Rochester Medical Center Medical Encyclopedia. Overview of Blood and Blood Components. https://www.urmc.rochester.edu/encyclopedia/content.aspx?ContentTypeID=90&ContentID=P02316.
14. EMedicine Health online. (2020). Kemp, S., Medical Author, Stoppler, M., Medical Editor. Anatomy of the Endocrine System. https://www.emedicinehealth.com/anatomy_of_the_endocrine_system/article_em.htm
15. ER Services, Anatomy and Physiology II. Capillary Exchange. https://courses.lumenlearning.com/suny-ap2/chapter/capillary-exchange/#:~:text=Filtration%2C%20the%20movement%20of%20fluid,is%20driven%20by%20the%20BCOP.
16. Cox, D. (2020). The Observer: Human Biology. Does the key to anti-ageing lie in our bones? https://www.theguardian.com/science/2020/jul/04/does-the-key-to-anti-ageing-lie-in-our-bones

PART TWO: THE GLYCOCALYX

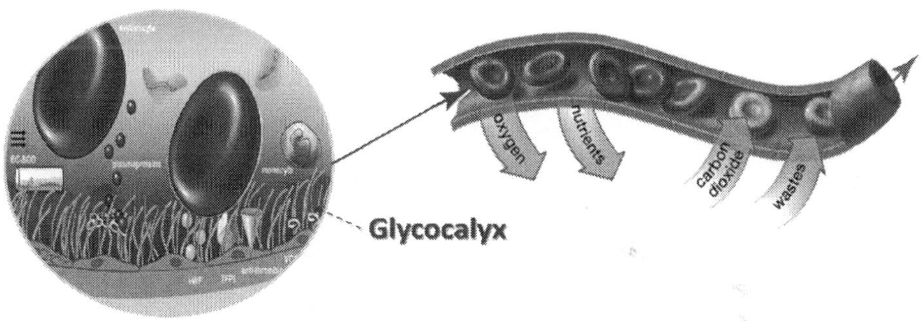

WHAT IS THE GLYCOCALYX?

Now that you have a basic understanding of the circulatory system and its components, let's turn our focus to what causes the breakdown of health. You are about to learn something that is the result of forty years of research and technological advancement. Very few people know about this - not even cardiologists! Here's why: years ago, researchers couldn't see the walls of the capillaries in detail, but thanks to the technological advances in electron microscopic digital imagery, we can not only see inside the cell, but we are able to watch as signaling molecules explode out of organs, each one being 100,000 times smaller than a grain of sand.

These technological advancements also enable us to see inside the body's microvascular system. We can now see and measure the activity inside capillaries as small as four microns (remember, that's 20 times smaller than the width of a human hair). When we look through these devices at the walls of the capillaries, we can see an additional feature of the interior of the capillary endothelial wall: a one-micron thick protective shield called by the glycocalyx. It is because of this technology, and the little-known glycocalyx discovery, that we can measure microvascular health and tell what extent the body has broken down. This knowledge empowers us to support optimal health at the cellular level and reverse or prevent the damage.

The glycocalyx is a dense, gel-like meshwork that surrounds the cell and the interior walls of blood vessels. Most animal cells have a fuzz-like coating on their external surfaces which consists of several carbohydrate molecules called glycolipids and glycoproteins. They are a combination of carbohydrate molecules connected to either fats or proteins that have a number of important function in the body, among which are cell to cell recognition, communication, and intercellular adhesion.[1]. The glycocalyx provides cell protection, particularly as a protection against cancer, immune system regulation, and plaque deposition on artery and capillary walls

The glycocalyx is a type of identifier that the body uses to distinguish between its own healthy cells and transplanted tissues, diseased cells, or invading organisms. Included in the glycocalyx are cell-adhesion molecules that enable cells to adhere to each other and guide the movement of cells during embryonic development.

The slime on the outside of a fish is an example of glycocalyx. The term was initially applied to the polysaccharide matrix coating epithelial cells, but its functions have been discovered to go well beyond that.

The glycocalyx is "a layer of membrane-bound biological macromolecules attached to a cell membrane or bacteria." It functions as a barrier between a cell and its surroundings. It also serves as a mediator for cell-cell interactions, where it protects a cell membrane from the direct action of physical forces and stresses. Without this protective shield, the breakdown of the cell membrane can contribute to the development and progression of many diseases[4].

Every cell in the human body has a glycocalyx, whether it is an endothelial, immune, muscle, blood cell, or neuron. For our purposes, we will focus on the endothelial glycocalyx which is this gel-like barrier attached to the membrane of each individual cell that lines the capillary walls.

It has various functions: it mediates nitric oxide synthesis and superoxide dismutation, acts as a protective "sieving" barrier (it only allows certain particles to move through it), inhibits platelet adherence and coagulation, and it regulates inflammation by preventing leukocyte adhesion (sticking) to the vessel walls[5]. If all this sounds complex, don't worry. we will explain each of these functions and their importance to overall health as we go along.

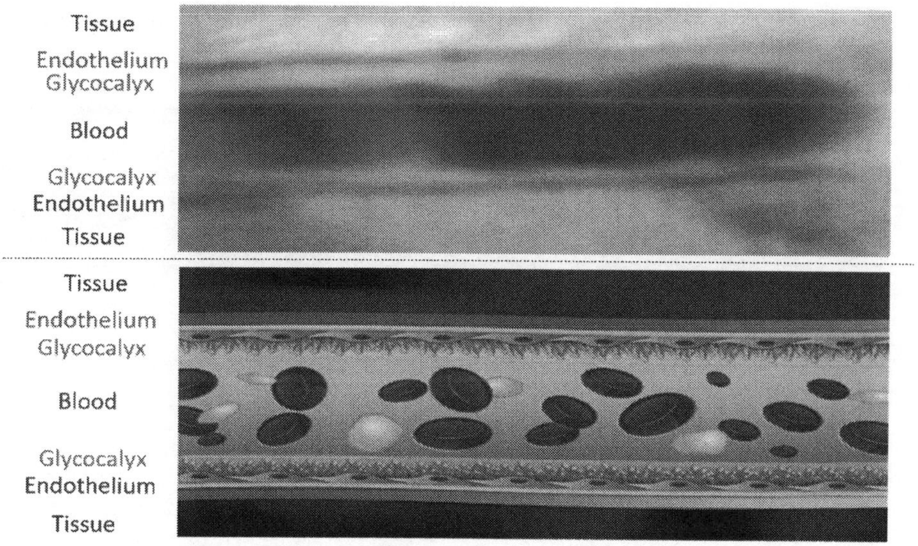

The top image is of an actual capillary at high magnification. The dark lines on either side of the vessel are the endothelium that marks the outside boundary, or capillary wall. The red blood cells (RBCs) are the blurry dots that flow through the lumen. They can either flow smoothly or sporadically, where you can see gaps in the blood flow. In a healthy vessel, the blood cells never touch the endothelium because the gel matrix is a protective shield barrier between the blood flow and the walls of the vessel.

THE DISCOVERY

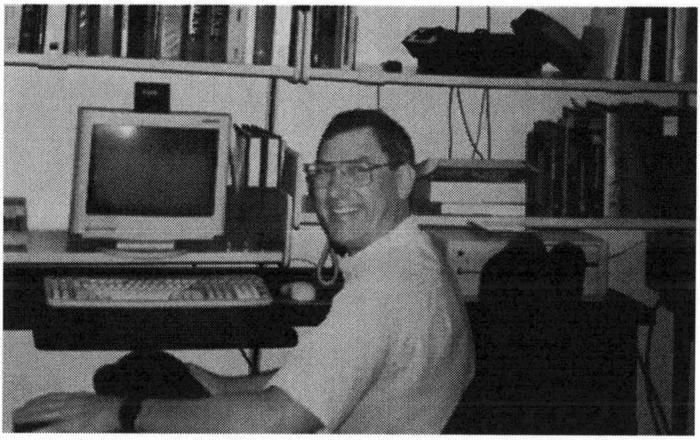

Professor Brian Duling, 1979

Scientists started using electron microscopes in the 1960s and that's when they saw the first pictures of glycocalyx. However, the pictures they took showed that it was very thin, so it was ignored and considered to be not relevant. The reason for this is because the steps needed to prepare tissues for electromicroscopy involve taking all the water out of your samples, and water makes up 98% of the volume of glycocalyx. So, if you take out the water, the glycocalyx collapses and you don't see it anymore, or it's very small. And that's why nobody paid much attention, and it was not considered of any relevance to the volume inside of the microvessels.

Then, in the 1970s, people started using light microscopes or *intravital* microscopes that allow you to look into living tissues at the capillary level. Dr. Brian Duling, of the University of Virginia, looked at living muscle tissues and noticed a suspiciously low red cell content in the microvessels. The reason it was suspicious was because if you take a blood sample from a large vessel and spin it down in a centrifuge, all the red cells go to the bottom and the fluid goes to the top, which is a 50, 50 volume fraction of red blood cells and fluid. But at the capillary level, there were big gaps between individual red cells.

They were estimating the volume fraction of the red cells by measuring the diameter and the volume per red cell. The estimates were as low as 10% or 5% red cell volume in the capillary tubes. So, there was a big mismatch, the large vessels, 50%, small vessels as low as 5%. This led Dr. Duling to wonder what was happening in the capillaries. Additionally, as soon as you start activating the muscle, then suddenly the red cell content could increase three to fourfold in the same vessel.

That observation of the low red cell content and the fact that it was also very variable led them to these questions. Was the blood diluted and the red cells were moving somewhere else in larger vessels, or was it that just fluid was moving through the capillaries, or was there something else occupying a lot of space? Was it possible that the space between the red cells might not be just fluid, but taking up by something else, like a glycocalyx?

The researchers started discussing what might be causing that. And Dr. Duling was the first to suggest that maybe there's something else inside there that is transparent and taking up a lot of volume, which he called a 'buffer zone' layer between the blood and the capillary walls in hamster's muscles.

Dr. Duling knew that there was this 'slimy stuff' on cell surfaces, (which we now know to be the cell surface glycocalyx) and so he put it out there as a hypothesis. Even though he had this hypothesis, they could not prove it with 1970's technology.

Dr. Hans Vink

Enter Hans Vink a doctoral student in Amsterdam, who encountered Dr. Duling when he began doing his PhD project in the late 1980s. His mentor in Amsterdam, Prof. Jos. Spaan, had been trained by Dr. Duling so, he introduced Hans to the hypothesis that the glycocalyx was significant in the function of the capillary. But in 1989, just two months after Hans started working on his project, Prof. Spaan decided to move on and do something else, leaving Hans in the lurch. The department chair told him that he could do one of two things: he could find another project or try to run the project without a mentor and develop all the techniques and build a lab by himself. Neither of those options appealed to him so he called Dr. Duling, who agreed to become his mentor.

For the next few years, Hans worked in Amsterdam and paid a lot of visits to Dr. Duling, who helped him build his own microscope and microcirculation lab and finish his PhD. After he finished his PhD in the early 1990s, the now Dr. Vink moved to Charlottesville, Virginia to work with Dr. Duling in his lab as a postdoctoral fellow.

DURING THIS PERIOD, THEY DEVELOPED IMAGING TECHNIQUES TO FINALLY, FOR THE FIRST TIME, PROVIDE SOME REAL EVIDENCE THAT THERE IS, INDEED, A VERY THICK GLYCOCALYX INSIDE THE CAPILLARY WALLS.

Those papers were published in 1996[1] and 2000[2].

After that, Dr. Vink moved back to Amsterdam and started training his own students. One of those students was Bernard van den Berg, who created the first electro-microscopic pictures of the full sized glycocalyx. He had developed techniques to stabilize the glycocalyx structures *before* taking out the water so it didn't collapse and could be photographed. That study was published in 2003[3] and it finally settled the discussion because now they had real pictures, leaving no doubt that the glycocalyx occupies a lot of space. Because of this technology, they can now study when the glycocalyx is small, when it's normal sized, and what the functional implications are for that.

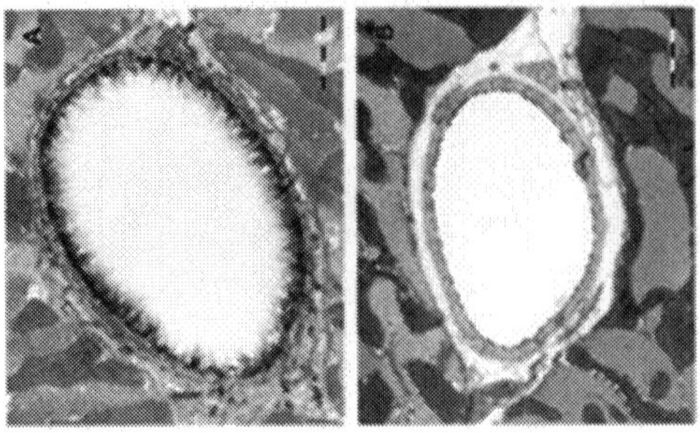

What Dr. Vink learned from this image is that the hairs of the glycocalyx stand up and become visible when hydrated, but when dehydrated, they shrink to virtually nothing, and become invisible. This image changed their understanding of the workings of the microvascular system.

These studies triggered dozens of other studies, which confirmed over and over again that the endothelial glycocalyx is essential to keep blood vessels healthy and that its damage causes:

- blood cells to stick to the vessel wall surface
- the leakage of fluids and macromolecules
- impaired endothelial nitric oxide availability

It also demonstrated that localized glycocalyx damage contributes to the accumulation of cholesterol and inflammation in the walls of large arteries at bifurcation sites in the process of atherosclerosis. This restriction is the cause of heart attacks and strokes. It was this, and subsequent studies, which supported his hypothesis.

After two decades developing glycocalyx imaging methods and studying the functional implications of glycocalyx damage by atherogenic risk factors, Dr. Vink developed a biomedical glycocalyx measurement system called GlycoCheck™. This system assesses the glycocalyx and measures microvascular health in a non-invasive way in healthy individuals and a wide range of patients with various health conditions.

THE CAPILLARY WALL

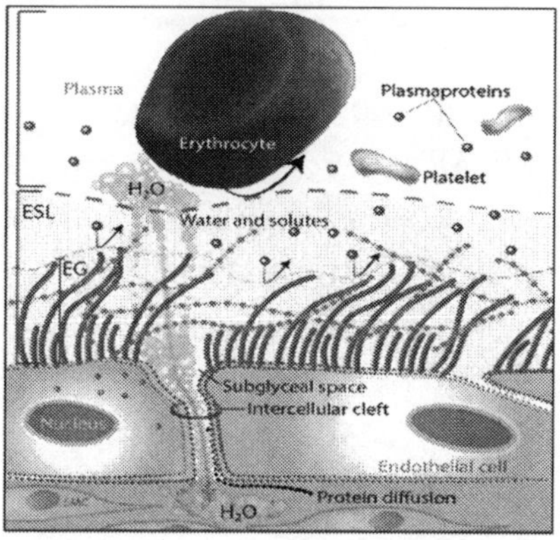

Let's take a closer look at the composition and function of the capillary using the above illustration. The blood vessel wall is composed of two parts:

The Endothelium (One Cell Thick)

The outside of the vessel wall is composed of the one-cell thick endothelium, which is one to two 10ths of a micron thick. The endothelium is composed of single endothelial cells that have gaps between them, called the intercellular cleft. This is where fluid passes from the capillary into the surrounding tissues. The cells look similar to shingles on a roof, which overlap a bit. Running through the center of endothelium lumen is the blood plasma that contains the nutrients, water, hormones, oxygen, and other constituents to exchange with the surrounding cells. A healthy endothelium lets the good stuff in and keeps the harmful stuff out. So, what makes the endothelium healthy?

The Glycocalyx

The glycocalyx is attached to the inner (lumen) side of the endothelium and fills all of the gaps in between as a continuous inner coating. It functions to protect the vessel walls from the blood passing through the blood vessel[6]. The 'hairs,' or bush matrix of the glycocalyx are composed of proteins and sugars called proteoglycans and glycoproteins. The words 'glyco', 'glycan' and 'saccharide' are the scientific names for sugars (these are not the kind that taste sweet). When you break down the structure of the glycocalyx, you will see that the sugar part of the molecule is composed of long chains of sulfated polysaccharides composed of single molecules called monosaccharides. Sulfated polysaccharides are special polysaccharides that are found in algae and seaweed. Glycans are either free glycans or are linked to proteins, which create glycoproteins and proteoglycans, or lipids, which create glycolipids. The glycans extend 1 to 1 ½ microns from the endothelial surface into the lumen of the capillary and make up 1 – 2 percent of the glycocalyx. The rest of the glycocalyx is the gel matrix, which is 98% water in which the 'hairs' of the glycocalyx are suspended.

The term "glycocalyx" is really an umbrella term for the entirety of free glycans, glycoproteins, proteoglycans, and glycolipids present on the cell surfaces and the lining of the vessels.

THE ANATOMY OF THE GLYCOCALYX

Cell Communication

So far, we have established that the endothelial glycocalyx is a protective shield, a gel-like, bush matrix primarily made of glycans that separates the vessel walls from the blood flowing through the capillary lumen. We also know that the bush matrix is composed of glycans. According to *Harper's Biochemistry*[7] these glycans make up the alphabet the cells use to communicate with each other. The Wikipedia Definition for glycocalyx is, '*A type of identifier that the body uses to distinguish between its own healthy cells and transplanted tissues, diseased cells, or invading organisms.*' This is extremely important to your health because the intelligent glycocalyx is not only protecting the flow of blood cells but is analyzing each cell that goes by to determine if it is healthy, needs repair, or needs to be attacked and destroyed.

Adhesion Molecules

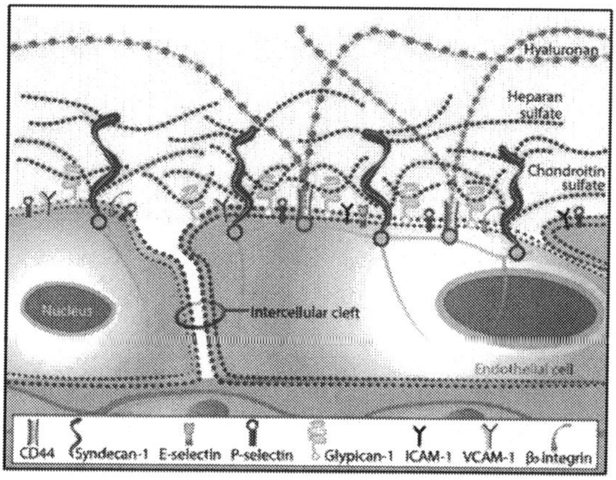

As you can see here, the long chains of glycans are connected to the endothelial wall. Under these, inside of the of this protective matrix are the adhesion molecules. They are molecules that react according to what is being communicated through the glycocalyx regarding protection, repair, or regeneration, to the cells as needed. We will be referring to the adhesion molecules throughout this section.

Interstitial Fluid

In both glycocalyx images you can see the intercellular cleft, which is a gap between the individual single endothelial cells. Here, the glycocalyx enables the exchange of nutrients and gases and communicates with the 'outside world' of cells. We know that water and larger molecules pass through the intercellular clefts while gases and smaller molecules diffuse directly through the endothelial cells. the exchange.

In the section on signaling molecules, you learned that there are many communications occurring between various parts of the body via the bloodstream. These communication molecules enter or exit the bloodstream and float around in interstitial fluid that surrounds the cells, just outside of the endothelial walls, looking for their receptor sites. This intricate communication network is vital for our health.

The glycocalyx is of particular interest to us in terms of understanding cardiovascular health. It plays a significant role in the regulation of endothelial vascular tissue, including the modulation of red blood cell volume in capillaries, which are necessary for the life-giving exchanges with the cells.

Shear Forces

The glycocalyx is continuously in contact with the blood stream. It responds to changes in mechanical force on the endothelial cells. Think about how the wind blows through trees, causing them to sway back and forth. This flow of the blood stream, called shear forces, acts like the "wind" on the "trees" of the glycocalyx and triggers the endothelial cells to produce nitric oxide. The force of hydrostatic pressure generated by the heart, means that as blood moves along the capillary, fluid moves out through its pores and into the interstitial space.

If you recall the section on the capillaries, we discussed how capillary walls are thin so that the exchange of substances can take place. The hydrostatic pressure in the arteries causes shear forces or shear stress on the blood flow in the capillary. Depending on the health of the glycocalyx and the hydrostatic pressure of the blood moving through the vessel, **parts of the bush matrix can break off and move into the blood stream, reducing the thickness of the glycocalyx**[8]. However, at the same time, exposure of the endothelium to normal levels of shear stress stimulates more glycocalyx synthesis.

How Thick is Your Glycocalyx?

Now that you know the basic anatomy of the glycocalyx, let's look at why it is important. While there are several factors that determine the health of your microvascular system, **the number one factor is the maintenance of the thickness of the glycocalyx bush matrix**.

To review, the bush matrix protects the cell walls, contains all the glycans for communication with the cells in the blood stream, creates the shear forces, maintains the capillary exchange, and communicates to the adhesion molecules contained within it.

There is a popular cardiovascular assessment called the Framingham Risk Score, which is used to estimate the ten-year cardiovascular risk of an individual. The Framingham Risk Score was first developed from data obtained from the *Framingham Heart Study*[9]. It uses an algorithm to assess the factors that can determine the likelihood of a heart attack: aging, gender, poor diet, lack of exercise, genetics, family history, reduced lung capacity, stress, high blood pressure, high cholesterol levels, smoking, diabetes, and overweight/obesity. **By the way, these are the same factors that will break down your glycocalyx.**

To measure how the glycocalyx correlates with the risk score, a study[10] was conducted in 2020 that compared the risk factors in 900 Framingham Risk Score participants with their glycocalyx breakdown. The researchers divided the subjects into three groups by their probability of having a heart attack in the next 10 years: 1) low 10%, 2) medium 20% and 3) high 30%. The glycocalyx breakdown in the Framingham subjects, correlated exactly with their risk scores! The medium-risk participants lost the use of 30% of their smallest capillaries and the high-risk participants lost the use of 50% of their smallest capillaries due to the glycocalyx damage.

THE PERFUSED BOUNDARY REGION (PBR)

Modern digital microscopic imaging developed and perfected by Dr. Vink makes it possible to view the glycocalyx on the smallest capillaries to determine its state of health by measuring the perfused boundary region or PBR. **The PBR is a reverse measurement of the thickness of the glycocalyx. In other words, it measures the damage to the glycocalyx or the loss of its integrity**. This loss causes the red blood cells to degrade toward the endothelial lining. This can lead to a penetration of the endothelium or unwanted activation of the adhesion molecules contained and protected by the glycocalyx. PBR is measured by the distance from the red blood cells to the endothelium – protection keeps it strong.

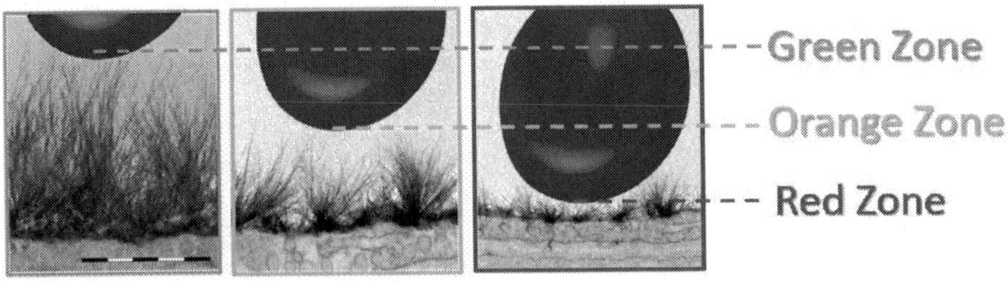

Green Zone: A smaller PBR indicates a healthier glycocalyx - less penetration, less damage.

Orange Zone: A medium PBR indicates a deteriorating glycocalyx – some penetration, some damage – early warning sign in need of repair.

Red Zone: A larger PBR indicates an unhealthy glycocalyx - more penetration, more damage - likelihood of eminent disease – emergency warning sign – in need of regeneration.

THE DOWNWARD SPIRAL OF CAPILLARY HEALTH

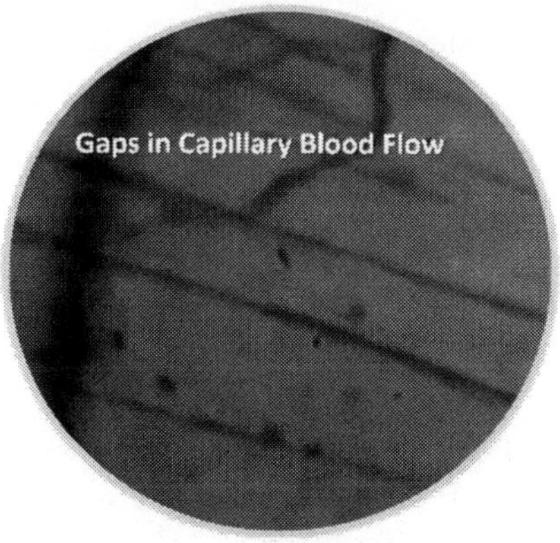

Initially, researchers who were watching the flow of the red blood cells (RBC), did not understand why there were 'empty' gaps in the capillary blood flow. Research has since shown that the glycocalyx controls both the flow of blood and these gaps. Right now, your heart is pumping an average of five liters of blood through your body; one liter of that blood is in your capillaries. However, by volume, there is twice as much glycocalyx (two liters) as there is blood in the capillary blood vessels. The glycocalyx fills all the gaps in the capillaries where there are no RBCs.

This creates what's called reserve capillary density, which means that more capillaries are made available on demand, as needed. To help you understand this, let's use a generalized example of what happens at the various stages of capillary health. ***Please do not take this literally.*** While we are using an example of flow rates and numbers of available capillaries, there may be more than three capillaries and greater or lesser flow rates.

Healthy Stage 1 – Warning signs

In the illustration below, you can view the healthy glycocalyx as thick lines on the inside of the endothelium walls of the capillaries. Let's suppose that in a resting state, there is a feeder vessel's blood flow rate of one hundred. The body does not need to access all of the available capillaries in the resting state because the demand for blood is minimal at rest. In our example, the blood flows through two capillaries at a rate of fifty each.

Now, suppose that you decided to jog. As your activity increases, the feeder blood flow rate that supplies your capillaries increases to 150. If your glycocalyx is healthy, the reserve capillaries will open up, so that more capillaries will fill the need for oxygen-rich blood. In this case, each of the three capillaries have a flow rate of 50. This configuration easily manages the volume requirements for extra oxygen, nutrients, and waste removal to the surrounding cells.

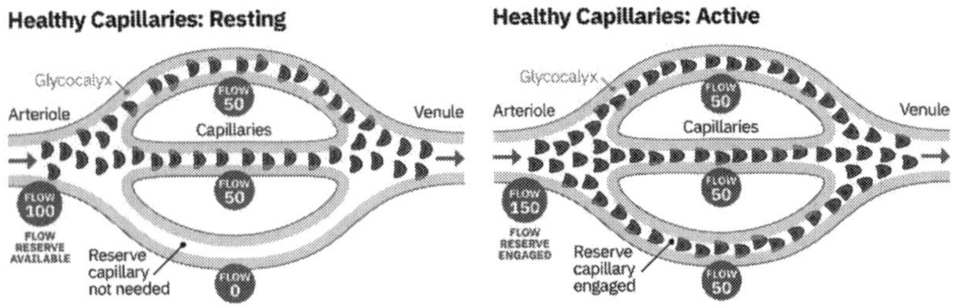

A healthy glycocalyx regulates the blood flow in response to metabolic demand for the delivery and exchange of nutrients and wastes, as needed. The reserve capillaries become filled with blood only when they are needed. In fact, the capillary density in an area can triple or quadruple within seconds! Capillaries can open or close to meet demand, allowing for perfusion. Perfusion is the term for the quantity of red blood cells in a capillary at any one time. It is the glycocalyx that determines and allows for more blood flow volume as needed to meet the demands of the body.

Unhealthy Stage 1 – Warning signs

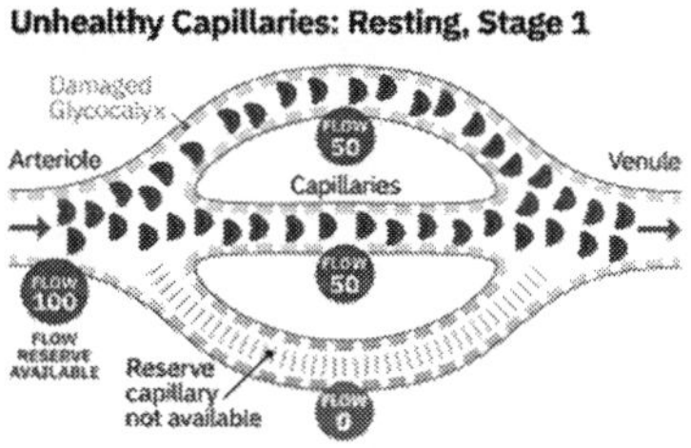

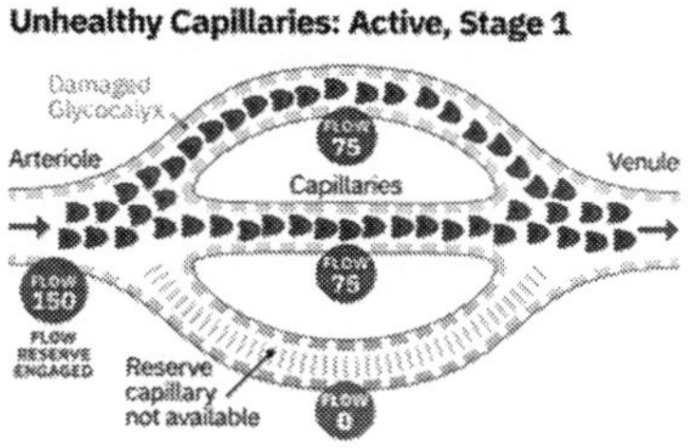

Now let's look at what happens when your glycocalyx starts to break down and becomes damaged. In these diagrams, the dotted lines on the capillary walls indicate slight glycocalyx damage. The strike-through lines inside the lower capillary indicate severe glycocalyx damage. In Stage 1, the organs begin to starve because they are either not receiving vital nutrients or have a toxic buildup of waste products. As the glycocalyx begins to deteriorate, the reserve capillaries begin to disappear.

As the illustration shows, assuming a feeder blood flow rate of one hundred, the blood flows through just two capillaries in the resting state. This is not that different from a healthy glycocalyx in the resting state. However, when there is increased demand, the blood flow rate increases to 150. But, because there is no reserve capacity, the blood will still only run through two capillaries, with a volume of 75 going into each. This is obviously not optimum, because the blood flows past the tissues more quickly and cannot transfer the nutrients or gases as efficiently. Further, the blood does not reach the tissues next to the third, auxiliary capillary, which means these tissues are not receiving nutrients or eliminating waste, and the cells and tissues will die. People in Stage 1 exhibit unhealthy early warning signs such a becoming tired and short of breath with little exertion. Life becomes heavier as they experience more early warning signs.

Microvascular Breakdown Early Warning Signs

- Cold Hands And Feet
- Leg Cramps
- Skin Problems Hair
- Thinning Fatigue
- Slow Wound Healing
- Lack Of Focus
- Memory Loss
- Certain Eye Problems
- Hearing Loss
- Poor Cardio Response
- Severe PMS
- Erectile Dysfunction
- High Blood Pressure
- Type 2 Diabetes
- Heavy Breathing

Unhealthy Stage 2 – Disease

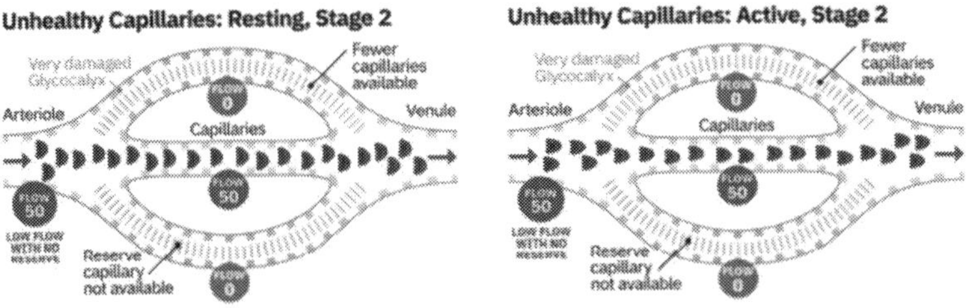

In Stage 2, the glycocalyx continues to deteriorate. In this case, there is no reserve capillary density and even fewer capillaries are available. This is due to a completely deteriorated glycocalyx.

Here, too, the blood flow rate is reduced, even in the resting state, because the capillaries are shut down and there is nowhere for the blood to go. So, even with a blood flow of 50, all of the blood would travel through just one capillary because there are no other capillaries available. So, anything you do to increase your activity, there is so much capillary damage there is nowhere for the increased demand to go and the capillary blood flow rate will remain low (at 50).

This is the state in which all the reserve capillaries are shut down. Cells are not fed adequately and there is a lack of oxygen and nutrients, as well as a build-up of carbon dioxide, wastes, and toxins. This leads to tissue and organ starvation, which then causes health complications.

People in Stage 2 can be extremely sick or even bedridden. They have trouble breathing and often need supplementary oxygen. It becomes an effort to perform even the simplest of tasks. They are well beyond early warning signs and into the early or late stages of:

Hypertension: blood pressure is higher than accepted level associated with loss of microvascular density increases the risk of heart attack, stroke, and kidney failure.

Diabetes: high blood glucose levels if damaged capillaries are unable to deliver hormones like insulin That regulates the movement of sugar into your cells. Eventually high blood sugar levels can lead to disorders of the circulatory comment nervous and immune systems causing blindness, kidney failures heart attack and stroke.

Heart Disease: insufficient number of capillaries per heart muscle fiber impairs heart pump function leading to heart failure. Micro-vessel blood flow to the heart can be impaired by clotting and oxygen radicals leading heart muscle stiffness, chest pain (angina) or heart failure.

Kidney Disease: breakdown of the kidney capillaries causes loss of its renal filtration system, causes leakage of blood proteins into urinary space, impairs production of urine resulting in hypertension and kidney failure.

Dementia: early cognition impairment or neurological complications associated with damage and the loss of capillary density in the brain to nourish and oxygenate cells essential to maintain an intact neuro vascular unit and support normal neurological function.

Inflammatory Disorders: an attack on capillaries by inflammatory cells result in damage and loss of capillaries. Increased capillary permeability causes tissue edema (excess fluid in tissues). Inflammatory disorders include rheumatoid arthritis, vasculitis, allergies, autoimmune diseases, and atherosclerosis.

Compromised Immunity: viruses and bacteria can trigger an out-of-control inflammatory response resulting in the capillary breakdown and unable to deliver nutrients and remove waste from cells.

Metastasis: weak, leaky capillary's allow tumor cells to enter the vascular system and redistribute to different parts of the body, causing tumor metastasis (secondary tumors). Healthy capillaries are more likely to contain the primary tumor and reduce metastasis.

Septic Shock: leaky microvessels result in a loss of circulatory blood volume, which causes a drop in blood pressure and impaired organ blood flow. This results in acute kidney failure, reduced lung function, heart attack, stroke, and brain damage.

Furthermore, whenever there is an interruption or restriction in the blood flow or the whenever the blood flow is restored after a heart attack or stroke—regardless of whether it is disease or surgery, there is substantial shedding of the endothelial glycocalyx. This leads to severe adverse effects, of course.

Glycocalyx Matrix and Adhesion Molecules

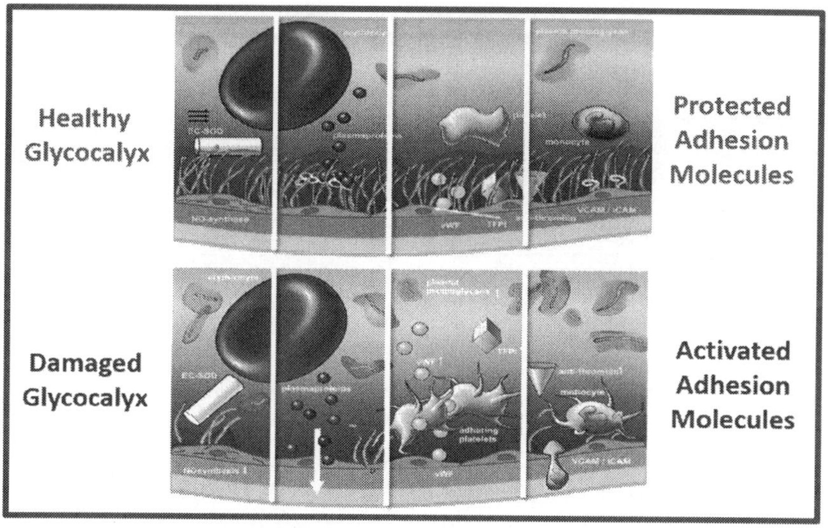

Let's start with this first image showing you what goes on inside even the smallest of healthy capillaries. You can recognize that this is a healthy glycocalyx because the bush matrix is abundant and the platelets, plasma proteins, and monocytes are floating above it.

If you look inside the glycocalyx you will see some items which represent the adhesion molecules that we mentioned earlier. These are not activated right now because they are protected inside the glycocalyx communication network, and all is well. This is the ideal state. The structure of the bush matrix is tall and strong, so its parts are functioning correctly.

The glycocalyx does much more than just help deliver nutrients and oxygen to the cells. It controls many vital bodily functions which are necessary for maintaining a healthy body. These include cellular communication, antioxidant protection, nitric oxide production, injury repair, immunity, and inflammation.

NITRIC OXIDE (NO) PRODUCTION

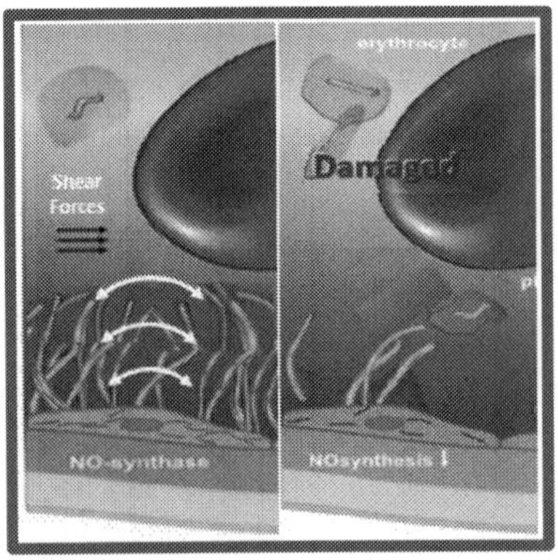

This illustration shows the relevance of a healthy glycocalyx and the production of nitric oxide.

Remember that the hydrostatic pressure caused by the heart pushing the blood through the vascular system creates shear forces. The straight arrows in this diagram indicate the direction of the shear forces. The bent arrows indicate that because of the shear forces, the glycocalyx sways back and forth, stimulating the endothelial cells.

Notice that below the swaying glycocalyx, you see the word, NO-synthase (nitric oxide synthase). Nitric Oxide (NO) is produced in the endothelial cells and distributed into the bloodstream because of this glycocalyx swaying action. NO Synthase is an enzyme that causes a reaction that produces nitric oxide (NO) out of l-arginine.

Robert F. Furchgott, Louis J. Ignarro, and Ferid Murad shared the Noble Prize in 1998 for their discoveries concerning nitric oxide as a signaling molecule in the cardiovascular system[8]. Dr. Valentin Fuster, who was the president of the American Heart Association that year, said, "The discovery of nitric oxide and its function is one of the most important in the history of cardiovascular medicine".

NO is an important cellular signaling molecule that helps maintain homeostasis in the cardiovascular system. It is a natural vasodilator that improves overall circulation. It keeps all the vessels elastic and helps control the regulation of blood pressure. It also helps control the hardening or calcification of vessels in your arteries as you age[9]. NO improves oxygen delivery to every cell and raises the effectiveness of your workouts. It is critical for neurotransmissions and helps prevent cognitive decline[10].

This means that nitric oxide production is failing because the glycocalyx bush matrix is no longer there to trigger the production of the NO enzyme.

A study published in the Journal of Geriatric Cardiology reported that a 50 year old women may produce 35% less NO than a 20-year-old, by and by the age of 40, men may produce 50% less NO[11].

When there is no nitric oxide production, the vessels constrict and become stiff, and so the red blood cells cannot pass through the capillary. As a result, the capillary shuts down and the cells and organ tissues are no longer fed.

Maintaining a Healthy Glycocalyx is the Key to Maintaining a Youthful Flow of Nitric Oxide Throughout the Microvascular System.

Antioxidant Protection

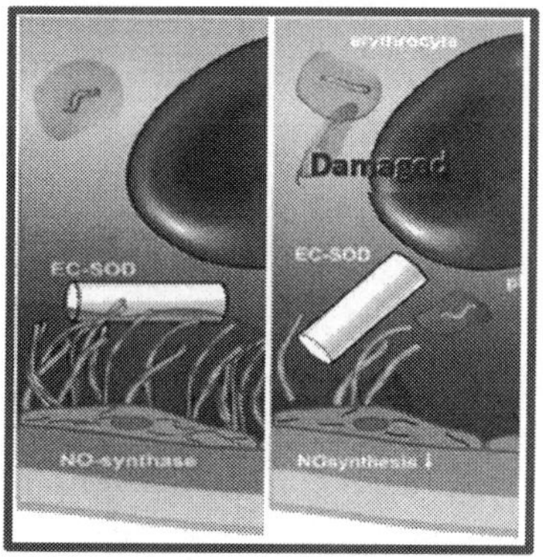

In this illustration, you can see a healthy glycocalyx on the left and a damaged one on the right. Notice that in the healthy glycocalyx image, the white cylinder represents an antioxidant called extracellular superoxide dismutase. (EC-SOD). This is a super antioxidant **and** is abundant in the blood vessels and airways. It the only known antioxidant enzyme that functions to scavenge biologically toxic O_2^{-} in the extracellular space[12].

Free radicals are metabolic naturally occurring compounds that cause damage to cells unless neutralized. Stress and exposure to toxins, chemicals, radiation, smoke, and other pollutants increases free radical production. Food-sourced antioxidants are chemical compounds that deactivate these free radicals before they can damage the cells.

The glycocalyx contains antioxidant binding sites that connect to these free radical scavengers. They float above the bush matrix like guards to ensure that oxidants (free radicals) can't get through and cause damage to the cells.

What happens when there is damage to the glycocalyx?

As it breaks down, the bush matrix starts to fall apart and float away into the plasma. So, the components in the blood, including oxidants, are no longer floating above the gel matrix. Instead, they are in direct contact with the vessel walls. The superoxide dismutase enzyme is no longer able to provide protection. The EC-SOD falls into the now sparse bush matrix and touches the endothelium. All antioxidant protection is gone. Oxidation begins eating the endothelium, causing a cascading effect because the surrounding tissues are not being fed.

As you can see, by consuming a high antioxidant diet, you can help maintain a healthy glycocalyx. A healthy glycocalyx will, in turn, provide protection against the ravages of free radicals and reduce your risk factors that contribute the diseases and an early aging process.

PERMEABILITY

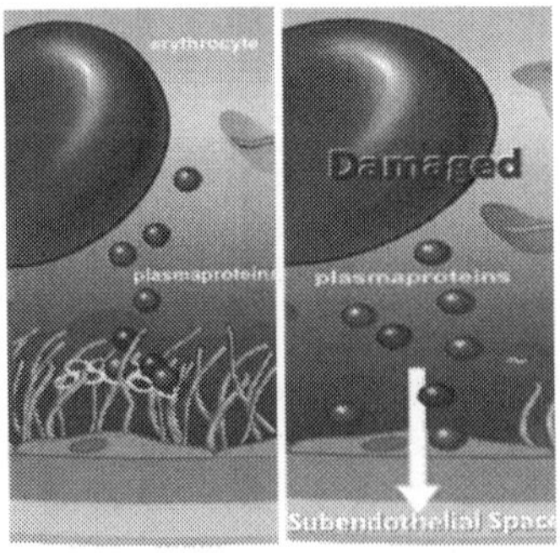

Permeability has to do with how easy it is for plasma to leak out of the lumen through the vessel wall. Typically, the glycocalyx acts as a protein-protective, selective barrier that keeps the harmful stuff out and lets the good stuff in. The term for this process is sieving. Think of a sieve in the kitchen when you are pouring your pasta and water into a sieve to remove the water. It works like that. Sieving keeps the water and the proteins separated

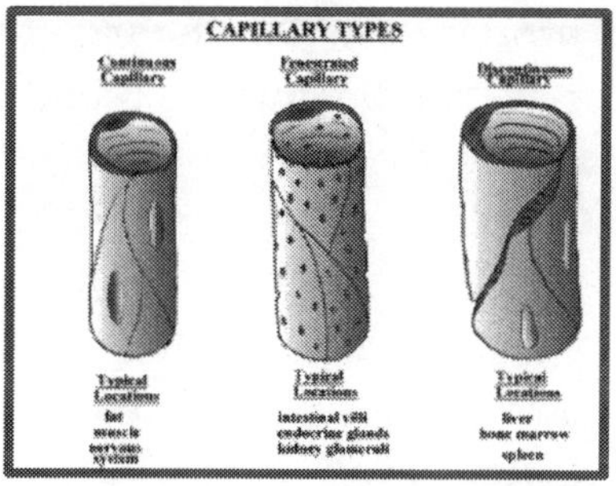

All capillary blood vessels are made up of individual endothelial cells that are only one cell thick. The endothelial cells are designed to facilitate the exchange of constituents between the blood and the surrounding cells, depending on the organ they reside in. For example, the endothelial cells in the brain have a very tight junction between them to form the blood-brain barrier. The liver endothelial cells have larger gaps, and the kidney or intestine endothelial cells are somewhere in between.

Permeability is critical to the function of the cell wall. A healthy bush matrix prevents large plasma proteins, like albumin, fats, and cholesterol from sticking to the capillary walls and filtering into the space under the endothelial cell.

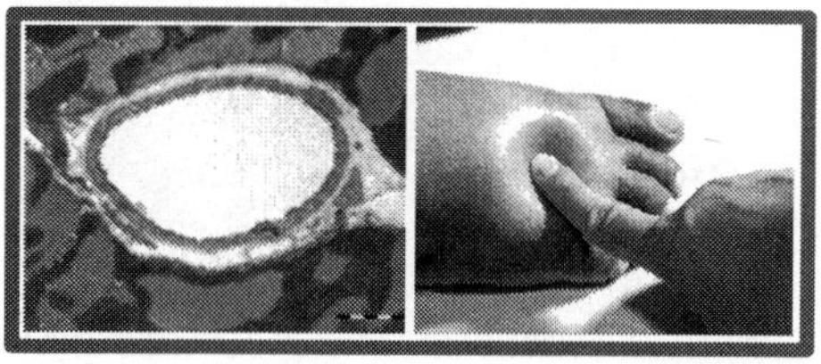

When the gel-like glycocalyx layer is damaged, there is no sieve barrier, so these proteins and fats, or excess water, will penetrate the capillary wall. When this happens, it becomes slack and weak, which then allows even more fluids to escape, causing a swelling of the interstitial space. This swelling is called edema. The glycocalyx is reduced whenever there is edema due to increased microvascular fluid.

When these fluids build up in surrounding tissues of the tiny capillary vessels in your body, they will cause the capillary lumen to shrink even more and then close off the capillary blood flow to the surrounding tissues altogether. This is the beginning of the cascading effect of blood pressure changes, oxygen and nutrients not being delivered, and the build-up of damaging free radical toxins that lead to organ damage.

A healthy glycocalyx maintains the proper flow of the right constituents in and out of the capillaries that maintains blood pressure, healthy cells, and organs.

COAGULATION

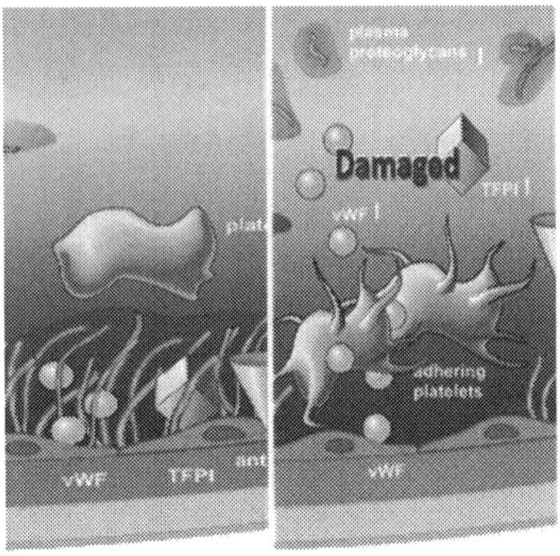

Coagulation is the term for blood clotting. Clotting occurs whenever there is an injury. As we have indicated, if blood flows too slowly and it starts to build up, blood platelets group together and stick to each other, forming a blood clot. Sometimes this process leads to problems, as you will see.

(The following is a simplified description of the biology of clotting. We are simply defining the terms you see in the illustration).

Normally, platelets flow along in the lumen, above the glycocalyx. In this illustration, you can see various shapes inside the bush matrix. VWF stands for Von Willebrand factor and TFPI stands for Tissue

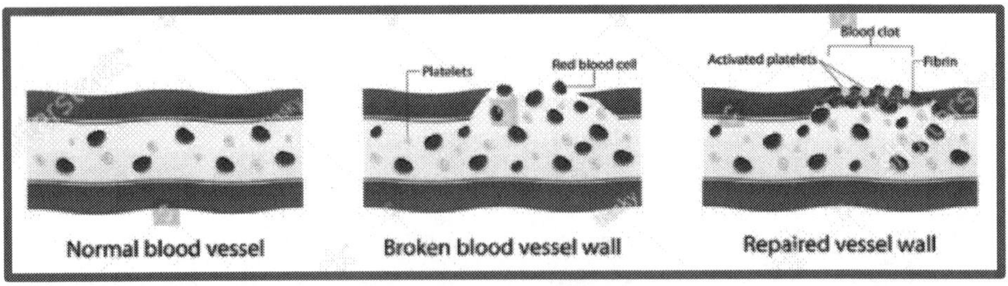

Factor Pathway Inhibitors. These are signaling proteins that signal the platelets to create clots. VWF and TFPI instruct the platelets to start making clots whenever the endothelium is damaged and

needs repair. They are encased in the bush matrix so they cannot touch the platelets unless signaled to do so.

In a healthy repair process, the platelets get the signal from the blood clotting proteins to repair the injury. The blood flow is diminished near the injury to reduce the risk of infection. However, the blood flow continues to other capillaries around the injury to ensure that those cells are being fed. This is a natural process and happens to repair an injured vessel.

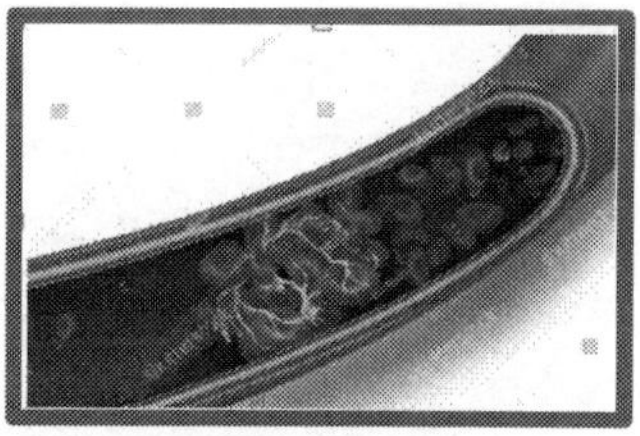

However, when the glycocalyx bush matrix breaks down, the signaling proteins are no longer protected from the platelets. Now the exposed adhesion molecules are constantly activating the platelets so, they are released and form local clotting within the capillary vessel. When there is no glycocalyx protection, oxidative stress and other risk factors cause injury to the vessel walls, which may trigger chronic clotting, in a process called thrombosis. This can lead to heart attacks, strokes, shortness of breath, dementia, leg cramps, inflammation, and if chronic, can trigger an overactive auto-immune response (the body attacks itself).

Immune Response

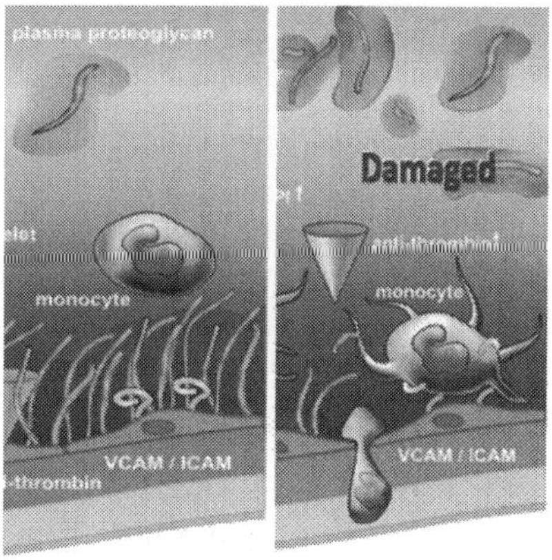

The health of the glycocalyx also impacts the immune response throughout the circulatory system. The illustration to the left shows a picture of a monocyte which represents the family of white blood cells. As you recall from the blood section, there are many types of white blood cells which patrol, protect, and defend against infections and disease. They kill harmful cells such as cancer cells and help other white blood cells devour and remove dead or damaged tissues.

An active, balanced immune system is one of the most important functions of the healthy glycocalyx.

The healthy side of the graphic shows that the white blood cells, represented by the monocyte, roll across the top of the glycocalyx. Here, they are in a patrol mode, hunting foreign molecules, infectious agents, cancer cells, and other undesirable particles such as inflammatory free radicals. Remember that the capillaries are constantly exchanging constituents between the blood plasma and the interstitial fluid to feed and cleanse the surrounding cells. So, while these patrolling white blood cells are rolling through the bloodstream they are, in effect, checking for any foreign invaders in the area.

The glycocalyx bush matrix is primarily composed of polysaccharide glycans whose function is cellular communication. When it is healthy and strong, it supports communication between whatever message is received and the immune blood cell's arsenal of tools that can handle the situation. These roaming white cells can effectively message the immune adhesion molecules to deploy the defense mechanisms of help, repair, or destruction to maintain healthy cells free from invaders.

This repair cycle, however, can cause inflammation. But, when the tissue is healed, the inflammation is eliminated and a healthy glycocalyx will regrow. Inflammation is normally a good thing, but it is bad when it spins out of control.

The damaged side of the graphic shows what can happen when the glycocalyx shrinks. First, there is a breakdown in the intricate communications which are necessary for proper immune function. As the white blood cells approach the endothelial walls, the immune-stimulating adhesion molecules activate the white blood cells to generate an early and repetitive immune response. This sets ups an out-of-control cascading effect of the various immune system cells that can degrade the circulatory system and cause auto-immune conditions where the immune system not only cleans up and attacks the bad guys but also attack itself.

What Causes Inflammation?

We have referred to inflammation quite a bit as a function of the immune response. But what causes it? *Cytokines* are small, secreted proteins released by cells that have a specific effect on the interactions and communications between cells. Cytokines trigger inflammation in the body. A healthy body can deal with these cytokine inflammatory events, but an unhealthy body may find them more difficult. According to a 2007 scientific paper called *Cytokines, Inflammation and Pain*[13], the goal in creating an anti-inflammatory drug or supplement is to block these proinflammatory cytokines.

How Does Inflammation Impact the Glycocalyx?

The inflammatory response is triggered by a decreased release of nitric oxide (NO) from the endothelium. This loss of endothelium-derived nitric oxide occurs within 15 minutes following traumatic shock[14]. According to a review in *Mediators of Inflammation*[15], the vascular endothelium is one of the earliest sites of injury during inflammation. The rapid loss of glycocalyx function is correlated with inflammatory responses such as diabetes, atherosclerosis, sepsis, and surgical ischemia/reperfusion injury. Whenever there is this type of severe damage, the glycocalyx sheds. Researchers have observed the shedding of the glycocalyx in response to inflammatory mediators like cytokines in the arterioles, capillaries, and venules under various experimental models of inflammation.

SUMMARY

The glycocalyx is a protective coating on the inside of over 60,000 miles microvascular blood vessels. Made up of polysaccharide glycans it provides an internal communication network which maintains the feeding, protecting, repairing, and cleansing of every cell in the body throughout the vascular system, down to the smallest of capillaries.

A Healthy Glycocalyx:

1. Facilitates the direction of blood flow to where and when it is needed
2. Facilitates the delivery of nutrients, oxygen, and hormones to cells.
3. Supports the removal of carbon dioxide and toxins from the cells.
4. Allows for the delivery of signaling molecules to specific target cells throughout the body
5. Facilitates the creation of nitric oxide from the endothelial cells
6. Holds antioxidants and protects the endothelial cells from free radical damage
7. Facilitates the repair of vessel damage as needed
8. Supports the balance of the immune system through the white blood communication network for inspection, repair as needed, or destruction of severely damaged or invader cells.

REFERENCES PART TWO

1. Noble, A.J. Drake, Vink, H. (2008). Hypothesis: arterial glycocalyx dysfunction is the first step in the atherothrombotic process. An International Journal of Medicine, Volume 101, Issue 7, July 2008, https://doi.org/10.1093/qjmed/hcn024.
2. https://www.glycocalyx.nl/research.php
3. Goldman, E. (2012). Endothelial glycocalyx: a new focus for cardiovascular risk reduction. Holistic primary care, news for health and healing. https://holisticprimarycare.net/topics/cardiovascular-health/endothelial-glycocalyx-a-new-focus-for-cardiovascular-risk-reduction/.
4. Möckl, L. (2020). The Emerging Role of the Mammalian Glycocalyx in Functional Membrane Organization and Immune System Regulation. Frontiers in Cell and Developmental Biology, https://doi.org/10.3389/fcell.2020.00253
5. Reitsma, S., Slaaf, D.W., Vink, H. et al. (2007). The endothelial glycocalyx: composition, functions, and visualization. Pflugers Arch - Eur J Physiol. https://doi.org/10.1007/s00424-007-0212-8.
6. Harper's Biochemistry, 31st Edition, 2018. McGraw Hill Publishing
7. Möckl, L. (2020) The Emerging Role of the Mammalian Glycocalyx in Functional Membrane Organization and Immune System Regulation. Frontiers in Cell and Developmental Biology, Cellular Biochemistry, https://doi.org/10.3389/fcell.2020.00253
8. Badham, J. (2019) Cells Under Stress. The UCSB Current. https://www.news.ucsb.edu/2019/019310/putting-cells-under-pressure.
9. https://en.wikipedia.org/wiki/Framingham_Heart_Study

10. van der Velden, A. van den Berg B. (Sept 2020). Unpublished results: Ggycltreat study – Leiden Univ. Med Ctr.
11. van den Berg, B. Vink, H. Spaan, J. (2003). The Endothelial Glycocalyx Protects Against Myocardial Edema. Circulation Research Originally published 13 Mar 2003. https://www.ahajournals.org/doi/10.1161/01.RES.0000065917.53950.75.
12. Jiang, Y. Chen, L. Chen S. (2018). Relationship between the endothelial glycocalyx and the extent of coronary atherosclerosis. Microcirculation. https://onlinelibrary.wiley.com/doi/abs/10.1111/micc.12504 .
13. Hunter, P. (2012) The inflammation theory of disease. Science and Society. https://doi.org/10.1038/embor.2012.142.
14. Zhang, J.M. Jianxiong, J. (2007) Cytokines, Inflammation, and Pain, International Anesthesiology Clinics: https://journals.lww.com/anesthesiaclinics/Citation/2007/04520/Cytokines,_Inflammation,_and_Pain.4.aspx
15. Christopher, T. A., Ma, X. L., & Lefer, A. M. (1994). Beneficial actions of S-nitroso-N-acetylpenicillamine, a nitric oxide donor, in murine traumatic shock. Shock (Augusta, Ga.), 1(1), 19–24. https://doi.org/10.1097/00024382-199401000-00004
16. Kolářová, H. Ambrůzová, B. Šindlerová, L.S. Klinke, A. Kubala. L. (2014) Modulation of Endothelial Glycocalyx Structure under Inflammatory Conditions. Mediators Inflamm. https://www.ncbi.nlm.nih.gov/pmc/articles/PMC3997148/.

PART 3
IMPROVE YOUR CAPILLARY QUOTIENT

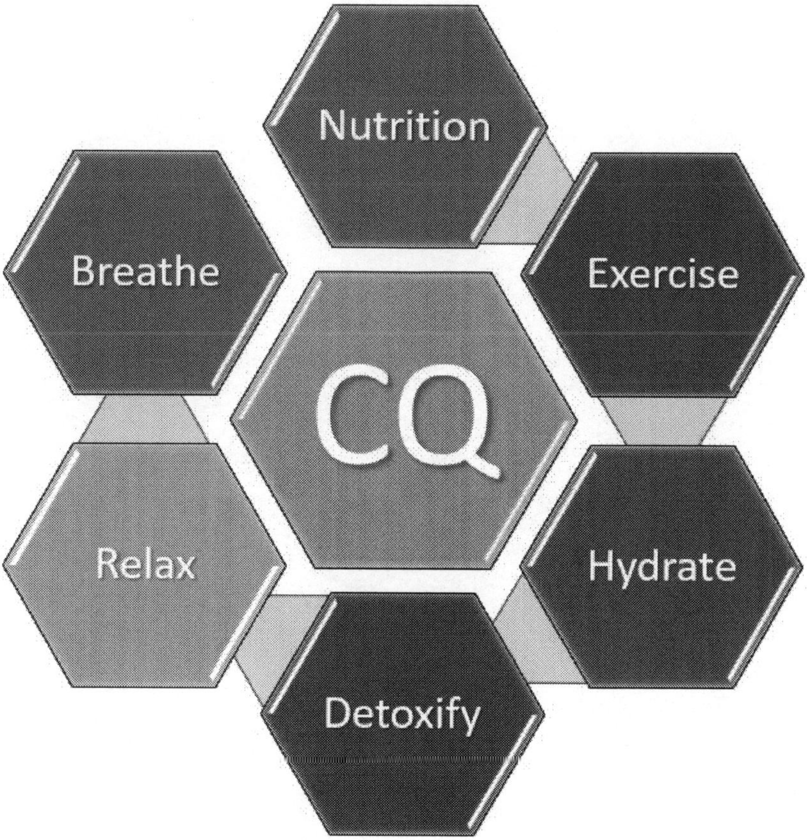

YOU CAN DO SOMETHING ABOUT IT!

Now that you have a basic understanding of the anatomy and biochemistry of the capillaries and the glycocalyx, it's time to take action to improve your overall health and improve your Capillary Quotient. We have learned so far that the health of your microvascular system is directly proportionate to the thickness of your glycocalyx.

You have seen the consequences of a damaged glycocalyx and, we imagine, are coming to the realization that taking steps to maintain and improve its overall health is imperative if you want to avoid the downward spiral into organ starvation and disease.

When you start to get the early warning signs—or hopefully before that—you can take action against the factors that damage the health of your glycocalyx to strengthen and rebuild your microvascular capillary network.

Your capillary quotient is influenced by several factors, some of which we can control and some we can't.

If you recall earlier, we talked about the factors that were used to determine the Framingham Risk Score for predictability of a heart attack. We also pointed out that these are the same factors that will breakdown the glycocalyx. They are:

- Age, Gender, Genetics & Family History
- Poor Diet
- Lack of Exercise
- Reduced Lung Capacity & Smoking
- High Blood Pressure, High Cholesterol Levels
- Diabetes & Overweight/Obesity

Obviously, we can do little about aging, gender, genetics, or family history. However, the science of epigenetics (the study of how your behaviors and environment can cause changes that affect the way your genes work) shows us that we can improve our genetic predispositions by being proactive with diet, exercise, detoxification, and lung capacity. These are the critical areas that you do have control over. To change your capillary quotient, you have to come up with effective strategies for lifestyle change of what you can control if you want to change your health destiny.

Lifestyle change is not easy. Why? Because, unfortunately, we are primarily driven by pleasure and social triggers more than by understanding and self-discipline. We are biologically wired to avoid pain. This is a survival mechanism. So, if it doesn't hurt, we typically wait until it does hurt before we make the lifestyle choices to do anything about it.

However, this is just a matter of perspective. With the right motivation and rewards, many people find pleasure in these health-producing lifestyle changes.

Social Modeling (Find Your Health Team)

One way to increase motivation and rewards is to have a team. There is a phenomenon in psychology called social modeling. Studies done on the effects of eating behaviors show that people tend to eat as much as the person they are eating with and match their pace. They pick up and put down their fork when cued by the behavior of another person. Also, the more emotionally close you are with that person, the more you tend to adopt their eating behaviors. As a result, people tend to eat 44% more calories when eating with others versus eating alone.

To become more proactive in your health, we recommend that first, you find and interact with support people who have the same health goals as you. It stands to reason, then, that social modeling can be used as a strategy to improve exercise and deep breathing compliance, as well. Find your allies so you can overcome your innate tendency to wait until it is too late.

You Need Motivation

There is an urban myth which states that if you put a frog in a pot of boiling water, it will instantly leap out. But, if you put it in a pot filled with cool water and gradually heat it, the frog will remain in the water until it boils to death. The allegory here is that because the change in temperature was so gradual, it didn't change the frog's behavior.

Just like the frog in the story, you can easily do nothing about your health until it's too late and you're in hot water. However, you *can* overcome this innate tendency toward the downward spiral of health. You just need to maintain an awareness of the importance of a healthy lifestyle NOW so you can avoid the pain and expense of the breakdown of your glycocalyx and its inevitable effects!

It typically takes years before the effects of an unhealthy lifestyle start to surface and, by then, it is often too late. At first you are young, healthy, and invincible. Over time, though, you may start to have vague aches and pains. You may go to the doctor and need to take prescription drugs. Later, you may get a heart attack or have a stroke. You may experience arthritic pain and need to have joints replaced. You may end up with one of those lifestyle dependent cancers. It creeps up slowly.

Many people are unmotivated to do anything about their health because they feel out of control. They are out of control because they don't have the knowledge, they think they need to make the right choices to be responsible for their health. As a result, they rely exclusively on their health care providers who even if giving great advice may be intervening far too late in the downward health spiral.

IMPROVE YOUR CAPILLARY QUOTIENT

1. Take the Right Supplements
2. Improve What You Eat
3. Keep Your Blood Moving
4. Improve Your Lung Capacity
5. Hydrate
6. Detoxify
7. Relax and De-Stress

MICROVASCULAR ASSESSMENT TOOLS

Before you start your journey to improved microvascular health, it's a good idea to find out where you are, currently. While a trip to the cardiologist can show you how much plaque or calcium you have in your vessels, you won't know what is going on at the level of the capillaries. You need a map to tell you where you are before you can plot a course to where you want to be.

You can do this through vascular imaging.

Vascular Imaging and Monitoring

Since discovering the critical role of microcirculation in numerous diseases, researchers have developed great interest in devices that can monitor the microcirculatory pathway. The early microscopes could not visualize the blood flow in the capillaries. It wasn't until dyes and digital imaging machines were developed to watch the flow of blood in these tiny vessels that doctors could actually see what is happening.

Today, however, some high powered cameras and imaging technologies are used to provide easy access to sublingual (under the tongue) areas that enable us to view the numerous capillaries of various sizes and levels of perfusion, which indicates microvascular health blood flow.

Detection of a microvascular abnormality is a key factor to start early therapeutic intervention in order to reverse microvascular dysfunction, to maintain efficient microvascular flow and to contribute to a better clinical outcome[1].

With heart disease, obesity, and diabetes on the rise, the medical professionals are constantly on alert for new medical devices, methodologies, and tests to evaluate the cardiovascular system, so that people can either stay clear of these conditions or slow down their progress. Today's cardiologists use X-rays, CT scans, MRIs, echocardiograms, ultrasounds, heart angiography, stress tests, and others to evaluate the health of our heart and vascular system and to act when they are not working well.

However, these tests—while valuable—are limited in their findings or usage in terms of preventive care. It is routine for people in late middle age to become familiar with one or more of these tests whenever they are presented with symptoms like shortness of breath or chest pain. By that time, however, the only solutions are ameliorative—drugs, stents, and bypasses.

But this is not just a concern for seniors. According to *Harvard Medical School,* as many as 4 to 10 percent of all heart attacks occur before age 45, and most of these strike men. It's a reminder that people should pay attention to the warning signs such as fatigue, poor concentration, ED, cold hands, and feet, etc. These symptoms could well be stemming from microcirculation and glycocalyx breakdown.

By the way, anything that increases blood flow throughout the microvascular system enables capillaries to open and perfuse to deliver nutrients and oxygen to the cells.

Anyone over 35 should get their microvascular health checked regularly. Early detection allows one to make natural, noninvasive adjustments for microcirculation improvements, the cornerstone of human health.

The GlycoCheck™

The GlycoCheck™ is the only device on the market that can accurately calculate your Capillary Quotient (CQ) the measurement of your microvascular health. It is the best imaging product and can record images down to the smallest capillaries with enough clarity to distinguish and measure their activity[2].

The GlycoCheck™ is a Class 1 Medical Device and **is unique** because not only has superior imaging technology that views and records capillaries down to the as small as 4-micron level, but it also has patented software algorithms that can measure and analyze the strength and the activity of the glycocalyx in the capillaries and provide the user with a Microvascular Heath Score (MVHS).

The November 2020 issue of MEDTECH magazine awarded the GlycoCheck™ class 1 medical device the Top Diabetes Solution Provider Award for 2020. To deserve this award, MEDTECH reviewed studies published by world-renowned research universities and hospitals, showing the effectiveness of tools used to both diagnose and monitor patient treatment.

At the time of this writing, the GlycoCheck™ glycocalyx imaging and analyzing software is being used in over 140 research hospitals and universities around the world. The research on the endothelial glycocalyx has been cited in over 12,500 papers. There are currently 78 published papers describing studies using GlycoCheck™ and more coming out on a regular basis.

These studies, using the GlycoCheck device, research the effects of glycocalyx health in correlation with many conditions such as:

- sepsis/septic shock,
- type 2 diabetes,
- early cognition impairment,
- syndrome X,
- stroke,
- kidney failure/hemodialysis,
- pre-eclampsia/HELLP,
- COVID-19,
- epilepsy,
- hypertension,
- atherosclerosis,
- heart failure,
- malaria / dengue, and more.

The GlycoCheck™ Medical device provides a Microvascular Health Score for the doctors and scientists to use as a way to determine the severity of the conditions they are studying and the patients' reactions to the treatments being studied.

Because this is such an effective device for monitoring the glycocalyx status and as a result the health of the microvascular system, a demand was created for a commercial version of the GlycoCheck™ medical device, which is now in the process of being produced available to health care so that they can analyze the microvascular health (Capillary Quotient) of their patients.

Microcirculation Enhancement Devices

There are a few tools on the market that are worth mentioning here. The role of these tools is to stimulate blood flow, which will reduce pain and improve capillary health.

The iTeraCare™ Device

Terahertz frequency waves are located between microwave and infrared waves. They are the same frequency as our body cells and generate millions of vibrations per second. The iTeraCare[3] device can either directly charge the body or charge water with terahertz frequencies to strengthen healthy cells and repair damaged cells while simultaneously expelling unhealthy cells. It enhances microcirculation and eliminates water retention in the body.

The BEMER

PEMF stands for Pulsed Electromagnetic Field. Devices that utilize PEMF technology emit electromagnetic waves at different frequencies that stimulate and encourage your body's natural recovery process. The BEMER[4] is a device that sends impulses in a precisely defined temporal sequence and generates a magnetic field, which stimulates the microvessels. With the help of this electromagnetic field, the muscle cells in the vascular walls of the microvessels are stimulated to contract, increasing the volume of blood that is pumped into the capillaries. This results in increased capillary density and blood flow.

The AVACEN

The AVACEN[5] is a therapeutic medical device and method that manipulates blood flow through the palm of the hand by using heat and pressure. The palm of the hand plays a vital role in the body's thermal regulation. It contains a unique heat exchange vascular network consisting of thick-walled large diameter venules. This complex arrangement of blood vessels distributes blood throughout the hand. It noninvasively infuses heat into the circulatory system, which then impacts the whole body. Infusing heat into the circulatory system reduces blood thickness (viscosity) and dilate the vessels to increase microcirculation. The heated thinner blood is moved throughout the body, relaxing the muscles and relieving pain, on its route to the smaller vasodilated capillaries (microvascular circulation) in the other extremities which the body uses to radiate the excess heat created into the cooler ambient air.

External Counterpulsation (EECP/ECP) Treatment

This therapy may be only indirectly addressing the microvascular circulation, but we feel it is important to mention it in this book for those whose health has deteriorated into the cardiovascular breakdown spectrum with artery disease or are in heart failure and are looking for a more natural way to rebuild their cardiovascular system[6].

External Counterpulsation (EECP or ECP) was invented at Harvard University as a treatment for angina pain. It has since become a therapy for multiple cardiovascular conditions. It is a safe, effective, and painless treatment used to grow new arteries (angiogenesis) in the heart and can also improve artery and heart function. ECP is non-invasive and uses no radiation, no surgery, and no medications. It is a rehabilitation alternative to heart stents or bypass grafts that are considered standard treatment for coronary artery disease.

The benefits of ECP therapy are: 1) increased blood volume pumped by the heart, 2) new blood vessel formation, 3) an increased flow of oxygen and nutrients, 4) enhanced blood circulation throughout the body, 5) increased nitric oxide production, 6) increased anti-inflammatory effects, and 6) improvements in systolic and diastolic blood pressure.

KEY SUPPLEMENTS THAT SUPPORT THE GLYCOCALYX

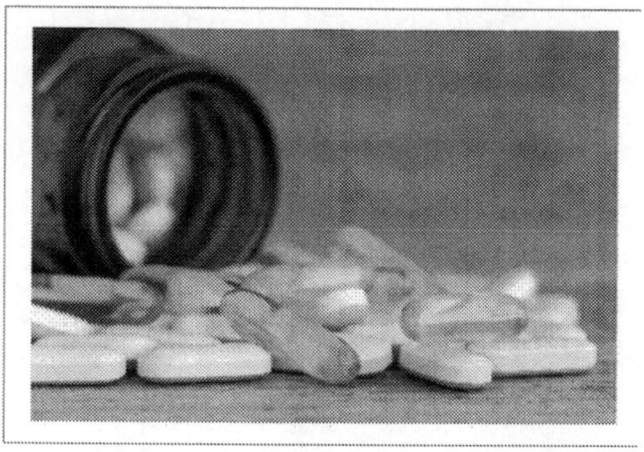

There are two primary reasons for taking supplements that support the glycocalyx: to stop oxidation that damages the cells and to provide building block molecules for the glycocalyx and the endothelium. In this section I will help you understand the benefits of a variety of supplements that will do just that.

You are about to read about a number of dietary supplements that have been shown to support the health of the cardiovascular system and the glycocalyx, in particular. I researched the ingredients in a number of excellent products to come up with this list. Now, years ago I would buy separate bottles of vitamins, herbs, and minerals. Then, I got smart and found products that have ingredients that work synergistically to support my health from companies that provide quality, tested products. I will also tell you when a particular ingredient is not beneficial because it has poor bioavailability. *Bioavailability* is the extent to which a substance is taken up by a specific tissue or organ after it is administered.

Before you make a financial commitment to a dietary supplement, make sure you are getting the best product for the money. If possible, find companies that have done double blind placebo studies on their formulas or have patented formulas. This means that they have done their homework and are products you can trust. Some ingredients in products are of inferior quality and may have come from countries where the air, soil, and water are full of toxins and heavy metals. You may have to pay more for better quality products, but you will know that you aren't wasting your money when you do this. Here are some things to look for when deciding if the product you are buying is going to deliver what it says it will: safety and standardization.

GMP Standards

GMP stands for Good Manufacturing Practices. This is a procedure that ensures that the product you purchase has in it what it says it does. Make sure it has been thoroughly tested so that you know it is not toxic, has a good shelf life, and has a valid amount of the active molecules. Prior to the Dietary Supplement Health and Education Act of 1994 (DSHEA), supplements were not regulated at all. Consumers were kept in the dark as to the research into the efficacy or supplements. The DSHEA gave people the power to do their own research and make determinations as to the benefits of a dietary supplement.

In the US, the FDA is responsible for acting against any adulterated or misbranded dietary supplement product *after* it reaches the market. Accordingly, manufacturers and distributors of dietary supplements and dietary ingredients are prohibited from marketing products that are adulterated or misbranded. However, that doesn't stop manufacturers from producing and marketing products that may not have what is on the label. Because of this, you need to be proactive in finding and taking high quality supplements from reliable sources.

Standardization

If you grind up a plant and you put it in a pill or potion, what do you get? That depends on where it was grown, when it was grown, what the soil and water was like, and how it was processed. Even from leaf to leaf or seed to see, there will be variation in the nutritional quality. You cannot count on something that is just ground up. You need to extract the active molecules. That means that in every bottle and pill, the nutritional fingerprint is going to be consistent.

To make a high-quality product with a good shelf life, manufacturers need to ensure that each dose is consistent from batch to batch. That is called standardization. There are a couple of ways that a consumer can be assured that the product they are taking is standardized. The first way is to know that the company providing the product has a state-of-the-art laboratory where the product is tested for consistency. Transparency in the manufacturing process is critical to the consumer seeking standardization assurance. The second way is for the company to provide quality assurance data from a third-party lab and other certified sources. Let's look at the various categories of supplements that have been shown in scientific studies to support the health of the glycocalyx and cardiovascular system.

The Classes of Supplements That Support a Healthy Glycocalyx

While I could just provide you with a list of supplements and their benefits, I would hope to educate you as to the classes of these various supplements, so you have a frame of reference for them. I have categorized them into the following classes:

- **Glyconutrients**: A glyconutrient is an amino sugar from a plant that mimics the molecular components in the bush matrix of the glycocalyx.
- **Antioxidants**: Antioxidants are compounds that inhibit oxidation. Oxidation is a chemical reaction that can produce free radicals, thereby leading to chain reactions that damages the glycocalyx.
- **Medicinal Herbs**: These are plants that have been traditionally used to heal dysfunctions in the body, which

are made from leaves, seeds, or flowers of a non-fruit bearing plant.

- **Other Nutrients, Including Vitamins and Specialty Items**. I have added a few supplements that don't fall into any of the above categories.

Glyconutrients (Amino Sugars)

Glyconutrients are plant-sourced *amino sugars*. These are precursors which are very similar to the molecular structure of the bush matrix so the body can readily convert them into the glycocalyx. Glycans (polysaccharides) combine with proteins to make the glycoproteins that help restore the protective structure of the glycocalyx.

FUCOIDANS (SULPHATED POLYSACCHARIDES)

Fucoidans belong to the class of glycans found in brown seaweed. There are many subspecies, and some have particular health promoting properties due to their percentage of glycans, which have a structure similar to molecules in the cell surface glycocalyx and the endothelial glycocalyx.

The various subspecies of brown seaweed have different properties when it comes to mammalian health[1]. Both the level and composition of the fucoidan depends on the exact species of seaweed and the harvest conditions.

As we walk you through the research, take note that the glycan molecules that have the most impact on the microvascular system are fucose (fucoidan) and rhamnose. There are two species of fucose in particular that are beneficial: *laminaria japonica* and *undaria pinnatifida*. A comprehensive review[7] of the therapeutic potential for brown seaweed provided a comparison between these two and other species. Laminaria japonica (34.1% fucose and 1% rhamnose) seems to have an affinity for the endothelial glycocalyx, whereas undaria pinnatifida (32.6% fucose and .4% rhamnose) has an affinity for the cell surface glycans that impact the immune system.

Laminaria japonica has been found to have anticoagulant activity but without the typical problems that come with blood thinners. A trial in mice showed that undaria pinnatifida fucoidan reduced blood clots without any increases in clotting time.

Fucoidans act as an anti-inflammatory agent. They promote something called "selectin blocking." Selectins are adhesion molecules found on platelets and leukocytes. By blocking the action of selectins, fucoidans can prevent inflammatory cells from invading tissue spaces.

They can also prevent the adhesion of platelets. What this means, in practical terms, is that they can help prevent post ischemic (after having a heart attack or stroke) inflammatory damage. You might remember that the glycocalyx breaks down during an ischemic event. Aneurysms, too, are partly an inflammatory condition. In one study, fucoidan reduced the swelling of an artery by reducing the number of inflammatory neutrophils (white blood cells) entering the area.

Fucoidans have been shown to rebuild a damaged glycocalyx. A study being conducted in Austin Texas[9] is using fucoidans to create therapeutics that mimic the glycocalyx. The fucoidans circulate in the blood and accumulate on the surface of the endothelial cells to restore barrier function in areas where there is atherosclerosis and vascular injury. Published studies have shown that the polysaccharide rhamnan sulfa*te* (rhamnose) can accumulate on the surface of endothelial cells and reduce inflammation. It can also prevent blood clots in the arteries during vascular injury.

Another benefit of fucoidans is that they are heparinase inhibitors. The body produces an enzyme called *heparinase,* which breaks down the glycocalyx barrier. So, certain species of seaweed not only rebuild the glycocalyx but also act as a preventative against this heparinase breakdown.

One study looked at the effects of brown seaweed on hypertension. High blood pressure can be caused by an increased vasomotor tone, a factor which determines the pressure within the blood vessels[10]. This activity is regulated in the endothelium by an enzyme called nitric oxide synthase (an enzyme that breaks down nitric oxide that we discussed in the glycocalyx section). The study looked at the effect of fucoidan on blood pressure and found that fucoidan increased nitric oxide production with a 'potent and persistent' reduction in high blood pressure.

In addition, a study on cognition found that elderly Japanese adults taking a fermented extract of the seaweed *laminaria japonica* for six weeks had improvements in both spatial and working memory[11].

AS FAR AS WE ARE CONCERNED, FUCOIDANS ARE THE MOST IMPORTANT SUBSTANCES YOU CAN TAKE TO SUPPORT YOUR OVERALL CARDIOVASCULAR AND IMMUNE SYSTEM HEALTH.

Polysaccharides (also called glycans) are structures composed of a base of single saccharides called mannose to which other single sugars attach while being formed inside the cell's manufacturing plant called the endoplasmic reticulum. They act as precursors which helps the body regenerate the gel matrix in the capillary and on the surfaces of cells.

MODIFIED CITRUS PECTIN

Pectins are gel-forming glycans the come from plant cell walls, especially from apple and citrus fruits. Typically used to detoxify the body from heavy metals, modified citrus pectin also has the benefit of supporting cardiovascular health.[12] Although pectins are not digestible by humans, modified citrus pectin can be modified to be absorbable. Modified citrus pectin inhibits *extracellular galectin-3*. Galectin-3 has been demonstrated to be involved in cancer, inflammation and fibrosis, heart disease, and stroke. Elevated levels of galectin-3 have been found to be significantly associated with higher risk of death in those with heart failure.

Modified citrus pectin can reduce macrophage activity, proinflammatory cytokine expression, and apoptosis, as well as lower inflammatory markers.

As a detoxifier, modified citrus pectin has been shown to chelate the blood from heavy metals. In one 2007 study,[13] researchers gave people 15 grams of a combination of modified citrus pectin and seaweed alginate for 5 days and increased it to 20 grams on day six. The scientists measured the amount of common heavy metals excreted in the participants' urine before taking the product and 24 hours after taking it.

- The results showed a 74 percent average decrease in toxic heavy metals without side effects.
- The amount of arsenic excreted in participants' urine increased by 130 percent.
- The amount of mercury excreted increased by 150 percent.
- The amount of cadmium excreted increased by 230 percent.
- And the amount of lead excreted in participants' urine increased by 560 percent.

Glucosamine Sulphate

You might have heard about glucosamine as a supplement that supports the health of the joints. Glucosamine is commonly used to manage osteoarthritis and joint pain but has had inconclusive results in that area.

The studies conducted to evaluate the benefits of glucosamine on joint health also found a surprising benefit; **the life expectancy of the subjects was increased by seven years with lower cardiovascular risks!**

A large-scale study[14] of nearly half a million UK adults was done to evaluate the association between regular glucosamine/ chondroitin supplement use and mortality from all causes. Results showed that consistent, long-term glucosamine with chondroitin supplementation was associated with **lower mortality due to all**

causes: cancer, cardiovascular disease, respiratory, and digestive diseases.

The subjects also had better lung health and lower cardiovascular risk because the glucosamine was producing a biosynthesis that builds the glycocalyx gel matrix. Aside from reducing inflammation, an animal study reported that glucosamine use can mimic a low carbohydrate diet, which could explain the link between glucosamine use and its protective effect.

Hyaluronic Acid – HA

Hyaluronic acid (glycosaminoglycan) is an amino sugar precursor that was first discovered in the vitreous body (the gel) of a cow's eye in 1934 by biochemist Dr. Karl Meyer. He discovered that it was this substance that helped the eye retain its shape. Then, during the 1940s, it was discovered that rooster combs are also rich in hyaluronic acid. Since they were more abundant than cow eyes, they became the favored source of hyaluronic acid for bakers, who used it as an egg white substitute.

In the 21st century, researchers are discovering that as you grow older, your body's ability to produce hyaluronic acid decreases[15]. While you can find HA products to help moisturize the skin, its benefits extend to the capillaries, as well. Hyaluronic acid breaks down in the acute stage of stroke injury. This effect is attributed to the enhancement of the inflammatory response. When HA is activated, it stimulates the production of new blood cells and perfusion of the blood in the capillaries is affected. This perfusion, called angiogenesis is critical for recovery.

Stabilized Aloe Vera Gel (Acemannan)

Most people have heard about aloe vera as something you keep on hand in your house in case you have an insect bite or a burn, but aloe has a rich history of helping your immune and digestive systems. More recent studies have shown that the active ingredient in aloe also has benefits for the glycocalyx and cardiovascular system.

Numerous studies have reported that aloe leaf gel (Acemannan) possesses numerous functions, which are attributed to the presence of polysaccharides, such as immunomodulation, antimicrobial, antiviral, anti-cancer, anti-inflammatory properties[16].

Antioxidants

Antioxidants protect the polysaccharides of the endothelial glycocalyx from additional damage and breakdown. Polyphenols are the most abundant antioxidants in the diet. These plant compounds offer various health benefits, as you will see below.

Antioxidants encompass a wide array of compounds that affect health. Your body stores its protective antioxidants in the glycocalyx gel matrix. Antioxidants neutralize harmful oxidative free radicals that cause this damage and increase your risk of conditions like cancer, diabetes, and heart disease[17]. Again, notice that oxidative stress (an imbalance between free radicals and antioxidants in your body) breaks down the glycocalyx protective barrier.

Most of the research done on the impact of polyphenols on inflammation and cardiovascular disease has primarily focused on the flavonoids. Flavonoids (also called bioflavonoids) account for around 60% of all polyphenols. Proanthocyanidins are a class of flavonoids found in a variety of plants such as red and black grapes, grape seeds, red wine, cranberries, strawberries, and blueberries.

Superoxide Dismutase– SOD

The primary antioxidant enzyme produced in the body and stored in the glycocalyx is superoxide dismutase (SOD). Enzymes are catalysts. In other words, they cause an interaction between two substances without, themselves, being changed in the process. We usually think of digestive enzymes when we hear this word but there are also enzymes that trigger processes in the body that have nothing to do with digestion. These are called metabolic enzymes.

The SOD[9] enzyme helps protect your cells from cellular stress caused by free radicals. Cellular stress can increase the process of natural aging, and levels of superoxide dismutase have been shown to decrease with age. Increasing SOD production may help protect or alleviate inflammatory, infectious, respiratory, metabolic, and cardiovascular diseases.

GRAPE SEEDS AND POMACE

While all proanthocyanidins promote cardiovascular health, oligomeric proanthocyanidins (OPCs) are of particular significance. They were discovered in 1947 by Jacques Masquelier, who developed and patented techniques for extracting them from pine bark and grape seeds. They have been used to improve blood flow, reduce symptoms of diabetes, ease swelling in the joints, and improve vein function to ease swelling. Grape seed and pine bark can both be taken as a pill, powder, or extract.

The polyphenols in grapes include resveratrol and some flavonoids. These compounds are present in the skins, seeds and stems of the grape and provide antioxidant activity. Grape pomace is defined as the pulp, peel, seeds, and stalks that remain after oil, water or other liquids have been pressed out. Because it contains the seeds, it provides the same benefit as grape seed extract

OLIVE EXTRACT OLE

Olive extract has been shown to improve cardiovascular risk in a number of studies. Olive pomace extract is rich in bioactive polyphenols. It is the byproduct of olive oil production, composed of the skin, leaves, and seeds.

Both the pomace and the leaves are included in the category of dietary polyphenols and have been demonstrated to modify blood pressure, endothelial function, and plasma lipids. The first study[18] here looks at the effect of olive leaf extract on blood pressure. Sixty males with a blood pressure between 121-140/81-90 were given either olive extract or a placebo daily for six weeks. The blood pressure in the olive extract group was significantly lower following OLE intake, relative to the control.

A review of the literature[19] about the benefits of the polyphenols in olive leaves to human health indicated that a considerable number of studies showed that compounds present in olive leaves, especially the oleuropein, are associated with hypocholesterolemic (cholesterol lowering), antioxidant, antihypertensive, hypoglycemic, and cardioprotective activity.

Researchers believe olive leaf extract can have positive effects on atherosclerosis, or narrowing of the arteries, which is the highest risk factor for heart disease. Elevated levels of LDL and total cholesterol are risk factors for developing this disease. One animal study[20] from 2015 assessed the effects of olive leaf extract on cholesterol levels. Rats who took the extract for eight weeks had significantly decreased cholesterol levels.

Olive seed extract has benefits similar to olive pomace. Another study[21] assessed the anti-inflammatory activity of a polyphenolic (of polyphenols) extract from olive pits and concluded that the polyphenols extracted from olive pits can both prevent inflammation and therapeutically eliminate inflammation.

Phenolic acids

Phenolic acids account for around 30% of all polyphenols. Compounds with phenolic acids are mostly found in berries, cherries, apples, citrus fruits, rice bran, passion fruit, mangoes, coffee, kiwis, tea, wheat, corn, and oat flours. One phenolic acid compound that has become popular in the past few years is *resveratrol.* The reason for its popularity is due to the so-called French Paradox. The French have been shown to have lower rates of cardiovascular disease than that of others in the industrialized world, despite eating a diet that is rich in dietary fat. Researchers have attributed this phenomenon to the fact that they drink red wine with their meals. Research into red wine revealed that the compound, resveratrol, could be the reason for their excellent health. Resveratrol has been shown in studies to enhance the expression of key antioxidants superoxide dismutase, catalase, and glutathione peroxidase in cardiac and aortic smooth muscle cells.

In rat studies,[22] resveratrol has been shown to protect against oxidative stress. This is because it is not only an antioxidant, but it can also up-regulate other antioxidant pathways in the body. However, in supplement form, it is often not bioavailable, and could reverse some of the benefits of exercise on aging, so make sure you are getting it from plant extracts and not from synthetic chemicals.

Blueberries

Blueberries have one of the highest levels of phenolic acids of the berries. Let's look at the effects of blueberries. Diabetics can have poor capillary health due to endothelial inflammation and vascular disease. A study[23] evaluated the effect of blueberry concentrate on endothelial inflammation in diabetic endothelial cells. This study compared the blood plasma of healthy individuals and diabetics for three days after being given blueberry metabolites (a combination of compounds known to circulate in the blood after blueberry consumption). They then measured the levels of endothelial inflammation. The researchers discovered that the diabetic group demonstrated a reduction in inflammatory markers. This led to the conclusion that blueberry consumption can improve vascular complications in diabetes.

Lignans

Lignans are another category of polyphenols. Lignans are found in various seeds, grains, fruits and vegetables, the highest concentrations being in sesame and flax seeds. The health benefits of lignans include a reduced risk of heart disease, menopausal symptoms, osteoporosis, and breast cancer. A dietary intake of lignan-rich foods can be a wonderful way to help prevent chronic illnesses, like certain types of cancers and cardiovascular disease. Flax protein, in particular, has been shown to help prevent and treat heart disease and support the immune system. A review on lignan intake from flax seeds found a 45% lower risk of death from heart disease. A study[24] that stood out for me was on flaxseed and its bioactive components. This study was conducted on menopausal women and showed positive effects of flax on reducing cholesterol and diabetic markers.

Another study[25] showed that adding 500 mg. per day of flaxseed to your diet may help protect against ischemic heart disease by supporting the relaxation response of the blood vessels and inhibiting the incidence of rapid, erratic heart beats.

CAPSAICINOIDS

Capsaicin is in its own category. While it contains polyphenols, it doesn't fall into that category, specifically. Capsaicin is the active ingredient in chili peppers that makes them hot. It has recently been used as a topical pain reducer, but it also has shown to be a benefit to the cardiovascular system. In fact, it has been reported to benefit obesity, cardiovascular and gastrointestinal conditions, as well as various cancers, neurogenic bladder, and dermatologic conditions.[26]

To show you just how beneficial hot peppers are, here are two large studies have been conducted to assess the intake of hot chili peppers and rate of mortality. One study[27] was conducted in the US to analyze the association between consumption of hot red chili peppers and mortality using a representative sample of 16,179 US, noninstitutionalized adults. The study reported that during 273,877 person-years of follow-up (median 18.9 years), there was a total of 4,946 deaths. The total mortality for participants who consumed hot red chili peppers was 21.6% compared to 33.6% for those who did not. The consumption of hot red chili peppers was associated with a 13% reduction in the instantaneous hazard of death.

Another huge longitudinal study[28] was done on 22,811 Italian men and women. The subjects kept a journal of how often and how many chili peppers they ate: up to 2 times/week, >2 to ≤4 times/week, and >4 times/week. During the 8.2 years of the study, a total of 1,236 subjects died. They compared the causes of death with the rate of chili pepper ingestion. **Regular intake was inversely associated with ischemic heart disease and cerebrovascular death risks.** They also noted that people with normal blood pressure had better outcomes than those with high blood pressure. They concluded that regular consumption of chili pepper is associated with a lower risk of total and CVD death independent of CVD risk factors or adherence to a Mediterranean diet. Cayenne pepper is a good nutritional source of capsaicin. You can purchase it in capsules, as well.

Nitric-Oxide-Boosting Supplements

Nitric oxide is an essential molecule required for overall health. Its most important function is that it regulates the dilation and constriction of the capillaries and plays a crucial role in the treatment of peripheral vascular and cardiovascular conditions throughout the entire body. As a vasodilator, nitric oxide signals the blood vessels to relax, allowing them to expand. This effect allows blood, nutrients, and oxygen to flow freely to every part of your body. But when nitric oxide production is decreased, the glycocalyx breaks down. Therefore, it's important to achieve and maintain optimal levels of nitric oxide in your body.

Nitric oxide production is essential for overall health because it allows blood, nutrients, and oxygen to travel to every part of your body effectively and efficiently. There are several types of supplements that can support the production of nitric oxide. Several dietary supplements are marketed as "nitric oxide boosters." These supplements don't contain nitric oxide itself, but they include ingredients that help form nitric oxide in your body. Two of the most commonly used ingredients are L-arginine and L-citrulline.

L-ARGININE

L-Arginine is a semi-essential amino acid found in meats, whole grains, and dairy products. Under normal conditions the body can synthesize sufficient arginine to meet physiological needs. Stress conditions, however, put an increased demand on the body for arginine so, dietary arginine is helpful.

Arginine is important because it is a precursor to nitric oxide.[29] It directly produces nitric oxide through a process called the *L-arginine-NO pathway*. As a result, arginine improves circulation. However, it is not very bioavailable, as a significant percentage of L-arginine is broken down before reaching your bloodstream. So, it may not be as effective a supplement as L-citrulline.

L-CITRULLINE

When L-arginine is converted to nitric oxide, L-citrulline is produced as a byproduct. L-citrulline can then be recycled back to L-arginine and used to increase the body's natural production of nitric oxide. In fact, L-citrulline increases the levels of L-arginine in your body more than supplementing with L-arginine itself does. Supplementation with l-citrulline has shown promise in lowering blood pressure in adults with pre-/hypertension. Studies[30] have found that L-citrulline increases blood flow, improves exercise performance, and lowers blood pressure. L-citrulline is considered relatively safe, and there is a minimal risk of side effects, even with high doses.

Artichoke Leaf Extract

Artichoke leaf contains compounds that can increase the activity of the human nitric oxide. It has been shown[31] to have antioxidant and other health benefitting effects. It may play a role in lowering cholesterol and thus help to prevent heart disease.

One study[32] sought to assess the ability of artichoke extract to stop deposition of fats on artery walls in rats with elevated levels of cholesterol. They studied rats in groups that compared the artichoke extract with and without a statin. Both sets of subjects showed a significant decrease in the concentration of serum cholesterol, triglycerides, and LDL in the subjects. The extract was proven to have a cardioprotective effect by increasing antioxidant activity. The effect of the highest dose of artichoke was more apparent than the effect of the lowest one. The researchers concluded that artichoke may act as a natural source for the elimination of cardiovascular ailments.

Other Beneficial Supplements

Vitamin K2

Vitamin K breaks down calcium in our bodies, and this property helps prevent hard deposits_(calcium and fatty material) from forming in artery walls. There are two forms of vitamin K. Vitamin K1 is involved in blood coagulation and vitamin K2 benefits bone and heart health. Vitamin K2 has particular value when it comes to blood vessels. A greater intake of vitamin K2 is strongly associated with a reduced risk of heart disease.

Vitamin K2 is found in dairy, fermented foods, and animal products. Several widely available foods are rich sources of vitamin

K1, but vitamin K2 less common. Your body can partly convert vitamin K1 to K2. This is useful, as the amount of vitamin K1 in a typical diet is ten times that of vitamin K2. However, current evidence indicates that the conversion process is inefficient. As a result, you may benefit much more from eating food-sourced vitamin K2 supplements. Rich animal sources include high-fat dairy products from grass-fed cows, egg yolks, as well as liver and other organ meats. The benefits of supplementing with K2 may be enhanced even further when combined with a vitamin D supplement, as these two vitamins have synergistic effects.[34]

Omega 3 Fatty Acids

Omega 3 fish oil is one of those supplements that has so much benefit for people that doctors often recommend it to their patients for everything from improved eye health to cognitive health. The evidence is overwhelming for using omega3 to reduce inflammation and promote blood flow.

In the 19th and early 20th centuries, mothers often fed their children a spoonful of cod liver oil each day. Think about the song in Mary Poppins about a 'spoon full of sugar.' That was about getting kids to swallow cod liver oil. It tastes terrible, but mothers knew that this one substance could stave off diseases rampant in those times. Their reasons were based on hundreds of years of folk medicine.

Rickets, a disease caused by a lack of vitamin D in the body, was common prior to the mid-1950s. The disease struck young children, which softened and deformed their bones. It happened to my aunt. She had a curved upper back throughout her life because of rickets. She was born in 1929, so they were just then making the connection between rickets and cod liver oil. Cod liver oil's connection with rickets wasn't scientifically proven until the 1930s. Not only is it rich in vitamin D3, but it is also rich in vitamin A (good for bones, teeth, and eyes) and omega-3 fatty acids. The reason why we don't promote cod liver oil anymore is that taking too much of it can be toxic. Cod can weigh up to 120 pounds, so large fish like these absorb a lot of heavy metals, particularly mercury. Fish oil from small fatty fish is the safer choice.

Toward the end of the 20th century, researchers began studying fish oil to discover its benefits as a dietary supplement. Unlike cod liver oil, fish oil doesn't contain vitamins A and D. But it's much richer in omega-3 fatty acids. In order for the omega-3 fatty acids in fish oil to work well, it's necessary to consume a fairly large quantity of it each day. Fish oil capsules make that easy. If you purchase fish oil supplements that also contain vitamin D3, you can get the additional benefit of a stronger immune system. Omega-3s are excellent for heart health.

The two types of omega-3 fatty acids found in fish oil are DHA (docosahexaenoic acid) and EPA (eicosatetraenoic acid). EPA and DHA can reduce the inflammation. Some studies have shown that these acids might also suppress an overactive immune system. An analysis of 17 studies[35] found that taking omega-3 fatty acid supplements decreased joint pain intensity, morning stiffness, the number of painful joints, and the use of pain relievers in patients with rheumatoid arthritis.

Balance Your Omega 3s with your Omega 6s.

Both omega-3s and omega-6s are forms of polyunsaturated fats and we need them both. The body cannot synthesize them on its own, so we have to consume them in the form of food or supplements. Although we need both, most omega-6 fats are pro-inflammatory so it's important that the right balance of omega-6 to omega-3s is achieved. An ideal balance would be 1:1. Unfortunately, our modern, western diet causes a skewed ratio of anywhere between 12:1 and 25:1. A big reason for this skew is that our diets are largely made up of processed foods, which contain cheap, processed omega-6 oils.

To balance out this disproportionate ratio and reduce inflammation in the body, we can reduce the amount of omega-6 we consume by limiting processed foods. We can also increase the amount of omega-3s we consume by eating more fish and sea vegetables, and by taking a fish oil supplement.

IMPROVE WHAT YOU EAT

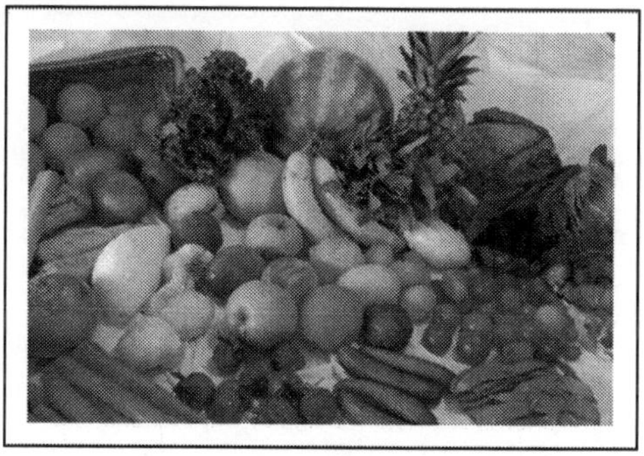

"Let Your Food Be Your Medicine and Medicine Be Your Food"

Paracelsus, who is the father of modern pharmacology, believed in the power of food for health and restoration. Most of us think we know what foods are good for us and which are not. Yet, most people are missing some fundamentals in diet that may impact the health of their glycocalyx.

Until relatively recently, we humans were consumed with getting enough to eat to survive—and that's still true for much of the world. However, we are dealing with different issues in the industrialized world. Food is readily available, so over consumption is our primary problem. This over consumption, as well as food processing, has led to issues with food allergies and sensitivities in many of us.

We are incredibly lucky to live in a time where many people's main problem is that of obesity because it is something we can change. It is not that true for many others in this world. Malnutrition due to lack of food is a worldwide problem, with three billion malnourished people, almost one billion of which are acutely malnourished. It may or may not surprise you to know that malnutrition accounts for one-half of all childhood deaths.

In contrast, the U.S., Canada, and most of the industrialized countries of the world, have malnutrition due to over-consumption of processed and refined foods that have little nutrient density. This is coupled with physical inactivity is the leading cause of death. These factors are a major cause of disability in seniors and are also linked to about 75% of total health care costs in the United States.

There is an abundance of low nutrient, high calorie food in our convenience and grocery stores, and because of the prevalent modern family structures, there is less of a focus on home-cooked meals and an increasing reliance on fast foods to keep our stomachs full. We spend approximately 90% of every food dollar on processed food. Yes, processed foods dominate our Standard America Diet (SAD).

Just because people know they should eat differently, that does not always translate into healthy nutritional behavior. Taste, texture, looks, the influence of hormones, and even the people with whom we eat drive us, biologically. So, making the right food choices can be one of the most difficult behaviors to establish.

Eat 8 - 10 SuperFoods a Day

In addition to effective supplements, eating SuperFoods is probably the easiest and most effective way to ensure you are getting the best nutrients into your diet. These are foods that contain important levels of the phytochemicals (micronutrients or phytonutrients) that have been shown to have an impact on health in a significant way.

• Apples • Avocados • Beans • Blueberries • Broccoli • Cinnamon • Dark Chocolate • Kiwi • Garlic • Honey • Olive Oil	• Oats • Onions • Pomegranates • Pumpkin • Spinach • Tea • Tomatoes • Turkey • Walnuts • Wild Salmon • Yogurt
Also unrefined coconut oil, kale, raw almonds, and algae/spirulina/chlorella	

As you focus on choosing SuperFoods instead of refined carbohydrates and processed foods that don't provide the body with good nutrition, your cravings will diminish, your liver will process toxins more effectively, and you will start to burn the stored fat you no longer want.

Eating Tips for Glycocalyx Health

- **Eat the Rainbow.** The easiest way for you to help your glycocalyx and your heart is to choose seven servings of fruits and vegetables each day. If your plate is full of brown and white foods, then add something green, orange, or red! Reduce the amount of animal fat and protein, as well as grains and refined carbohydrates.
- Just like Mama said, **eat your vegetables**. Eat a variety of fresh, live foods. There is a sound reason for creating a variety of foods in your diet. Even if you overeat simple, wonderful foods, you can develop an allergy to them. Further, if you don't eat a variety of foods, especially those that are in season,

then you may deprive yourself of the nutrients that you need. So, it is important to be sure to eat seasonal foods.

- **Eat regularly**. Many of us eat three meals a day but you may want to eat five meals a day that have smaller portions at each meal so you will get a steady burn throughout the day and eliminate cravings and the ups and downs in energy that you often get.
- **Do not skip meals** unless you are practicing intermittent fasting. Skipping meals can throw off your energy levels and cause your blood sugar to drop. Breakfast is one of the most important meals of the day because it sets you up for the entire day for energy management and a good steady burn.
- **Eat the same relative number of calories at each meal**. Often people will eat two tiny meals and then the pig out on one giant meal at dinnertime. What happens then is that your body feels bogged down, trying to digest that one giant meal and, what doesn't get burned, converts to fat.

KEEP YOUR BLOOD MOVING

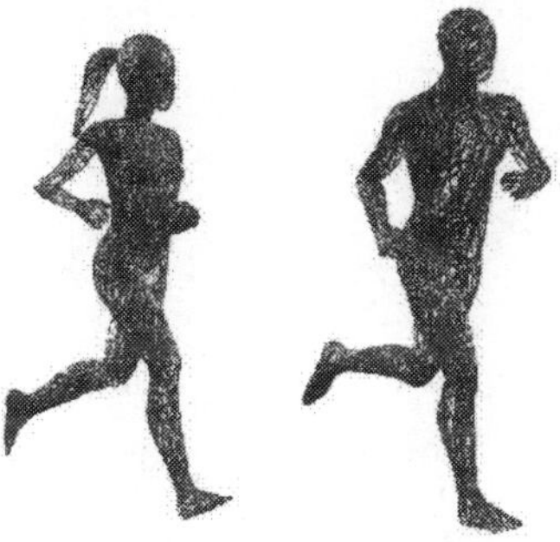

Studies have shown that increasing your microcirculation can help enhance the delivery of oxygen and nutrition to the muscles while helping to carry away toxins. The result is a healthier glycocalyx throughout your body. Earlier we alluded to the power of exercise in maintaining a healthy glycocalyx. Exercise increases shear stress, which keeps blood vessels open, and capillaries perfused. It reduces your risk for high blood pressure, elevated LDL, memory problems, and heart attacks. These are huge reasons to keep us motivated to exercise!

Although we might not like to confront it, exercise is the number one thing we can do to help maintain good circulation and promote health. Just like any other proactive health strategy, starting an exercise program is hard. Our muscles ache. Our old injuries might re-surface. We have to take time away from the things that might actually interest us to do it. And, worse yet, maintaining an exercise program is even harder! If we get past the initial soreness and into a routine, we can still be blocked by life getting in the way. One or two days goes by and we don't go back to the gym or stop doing our exercises and it becomes much harder to start again.

It is particularly difficult to maintain an exercise program if it is something you don't enjoy. The trick is to find something you *do* enjoy. You might be motivated by a class, a sport, or dance instead of going to the gym. You might like competition and choose someone to compare notes with. You might even like taking daily walks with your dog or best friend. Find the thing that will help you maintain your exercise program so that you can avoid the pain and deterioration that will happen if you don't.

What Happens if You Don't Exercise?

Let's look at some of the consequences of not maintaining an exercise regimen. It will come as no surprise to you that the majority of us sit too much. One significant study[36] that followed 222,497 Australian adults for several years, found that those who sat for 11 hours a day or more were at the highest risk of all-cause mortality, followed by those who sat for 8 to 11 hours per day.

You think that eleven hours a day is a lot? Think about it; many of us do that in this day and age. We sit to eat. We sit to drive. We sit to work. We sit to watch television. We sit to read. We sit to go to meetings. We sit at church. Sitting too much can lead to health problems, so we have to get off our butts and move or at least stand!

One reason that not moving is so averse to maintaining health is that if you aren't building muscle as you age, you are going to gain weight unless you reduce how much you eat. We lose an average of 5% of muscle mass every ten years after the age of thirty-five unless we intentionally work on strength training.

How Exercise Increases Your Capillary Quotient

There is growing evidence that diseases with an inflammatory component can be treated through physical exercise. A multi-agency US study looked in detail at 45 articles published between 1950 and 2011 that relate physical activity, cancer survival and biomarkers potentially relevant to cancer. There was consistent evidence **from 27 of the**

studies that physical activity reduced mortality from breast and colon cancers of all causes[37].

In addition, the *type* of exercise may have an influence over how well it can support your health. High-intensity Interval Training (HIIT) is known to improve health-related fitness in general and lifestyle-induced chronic diseases by protecting the microvasculature, including the glycocalyx barrier. A study[38] that measured the glycocalyx to detect exercise-induced changes, showed a correlation between maximal exercise performance capacity and glycocalyx thickness (determined by perfused boundary region). Increased exercise performance at follow-up also correlated with glycocalyx thickness and increased high-intensity sprinting speed was associated with an increased number of perfused vessels.

The Three Critical Forms of Exercise

It is important to move your body in three ways to maintain your health:

- Flexibility Activities stretch or loosen muscles and joints and help with balance and coordination. Do these slowly, holding each stretch. Many of us will go work out, go to the gym, and do aerobics but we don't take the time to stretch. You have to focus on maintaining balance as you get older. So, stretch slowly and breathe. This is the best way to keep your muscles and joints flexible. Spend five minutes per day stretching.
-
- Strengthening activities make your muscles and bones stronger by working them harder. This is usually done against resistance, and it also helps with balance and coordination. The other concern we have is the risk for osteoporosis (brittle, weak bones). Remember, bones send out signaling molecules improve memory and increase longevity. Weight bearing exercises keep your bones strong. Just doing aerobics is not

enough. You need to do your lifting, your push-ups, and your sit-ups—anything that continues to keep your muscles strong. Even using a mini trampoline will help strengthen your muscles, organs, and bones. Spend at least 30 minutes per week strengthening.

- Endurance or Aerobic Activities can be anything that makes you feel good and increases your respiratory rate. You can walk, go swimming, bike, go dancing, or anything else that causes you to breathe more deeply and quickly. A minimum goal for aerobic activity is 120 minutes each week, or 20 minutes, 4 times a week.

IMPROVE YOUR LUNG CAPACITY

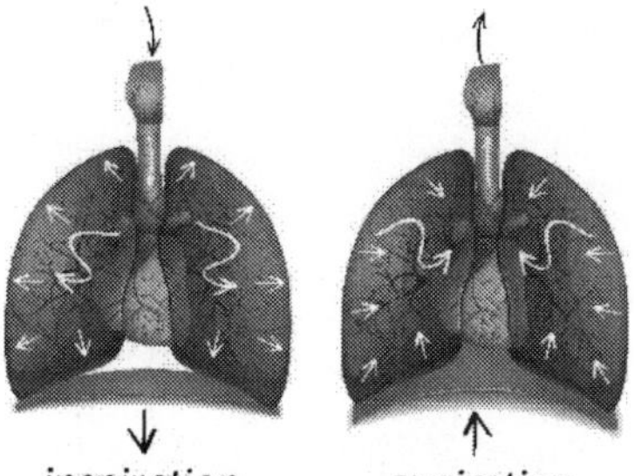

If you do nothing else as a result of reading this book than improving your breathing, you will be way ahead of the game. Most of us don't think about the power of breathing to reverse and prevent negative health outcomes. The famous Framingham Study[39] (which followed 5,200 individuals for three decades) showed that **the greatest predictor of health and longevity is lung volume.** People with greater lung capacity were healthier and lived longer than those with decreased lung capacity.

Our lung capacity begins to decrease around age thirty. Lung capacity drops 9 to 22% every decade after that, so by the time we are fifty, our lung capacity may be half of what it was when we were children. Decreased lung capacity means that less oxygen is getting into our cells. Evidence of reduced lung capacity is shortness of breath, decreased endurance, and susceptibility to respiratory illness.

The better you can breathe the better health you have. It's as simple as that. We find that this is one of the easiest habits to integrate into your life. You will experience immediate benefits from increased breathing capacity and will notice that you are more relaxed and alert.

Deep breathing also enables you to eliminate the buildup of stress hormones. Stress hormones, primarily cortisol, build up in your body and contribute to a number of negative outcomes, including anxiety, depression, and inflammation, unless you eliminate them through breathing. When you practice twenty minutes of deep breathing you will eliminate the excess cortisol levels in your bloodstream and bring your body back into balance. So, breathing is critical to maintaining optimum health and well-being.

Of course, any activity like lap swimming, HIIT, jogging, playing a wind instrument, singing, or hatha yoga will automatically improve your lung capacity but in addition there are many other opportunities to practice deliberate breathing:

- In the morning before you get out of bed.
- At stop lights
- While taking a shower
- Sitting at the computer
- Lying in bed before sleep (10 deep, slow breaths will help you sleep)
- While in the bathroom, before you get ready to leave.
- When checking your emails
- Before you get out of bed in the morning
- While watching TV
- When stretching

Deep Breathing

- 3 Minutes to Break a Stress Cycle
- 10 Minutes to Remove ½ of your Stress Hormones.
- 20 Minutes to Create Endorphins

HYDRATE EFFECTIVELY

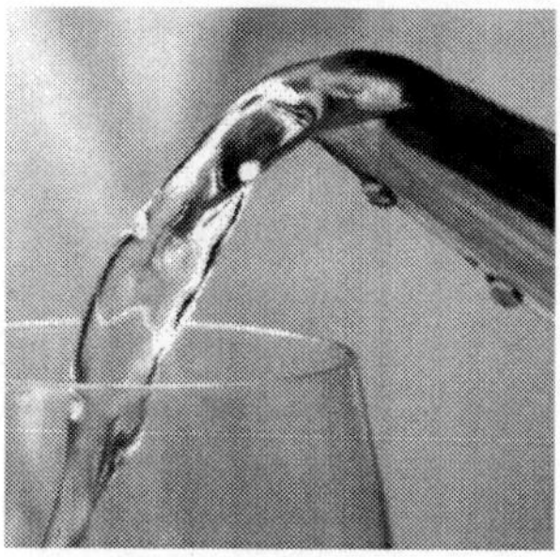

Remember that the glycocalyx is 98% water! Hydration is very important in maintaining the fluid levels in your body, from your skin to your capillaries. Further, it turns out that water enhanced with dissolved hydrogen has extremely beneficial effects on the endothelium, as well as on cognition and other important areas of health.

We all know that it is important to drink water. More than 50 percent of the human body is made of water. Our brains and hearts are 73 percent water, and our lungs are 83 percent water. Blood plasma is over 90 percent water.

Drinking water helps maintain our balance of body fluids. It lubricates the cells and systems, and also keeps your skin and eyes moist. Cells that do not maintain their balance of fluids and electrolytes will shrivel. When muscle cells don't have adequate fluids, they do not work as well, and performance can suffer. And—most importantly—water impacts the viscosity of blood and even impacts the health and integrity of your glycocalyx.

So, even though we know that it is important to drink water, many of us don't do it. A study on American water-drinking habits was conducted by a researcher at the Centers of Disease Control showing that only ten percent of Americans drink water every day[40]! It is amazing, knowing the importance of water at the number of people who will say that they don't drink it because they don't like the taste. Instead, they will opt for soda pop or some other form of flavored liquid, like coffee, thinking they are hydrating when in fact they are dehydrating.

One of the most important reasons to stay hydrated is because the glycocalyx is 98% water. Now, remember that the endothelium enables fluids to move easily from the blood to the tissue. When the glycocalyx dehydrates, it essentially disappears[41], and unwanted substances can penetrate the barrier and enter the tissues and organs. So, it is essential for the glycocalyx to be hydrated.

How Much Water Should I Drink?

Although there are no hard and fast rules, a favorite goal is 50% of your body weight in ounces of water. (130 lbs. = 65 oz. = 8 x 8 oz. glasses). Some people do not need this much water to be fully hydrated. In fact, over-drinking water can reduce your blood sodium levels. Very few people will overly hydrate themselves. The best way to tell if you are getting enough water is to drink enough water throughout the day to produce light-colored urine.

If you don't like the taste of water, use non-caffeinated herbal teas and do not use synthetic sweeteners. We like to add fresh lemon juice, slices of cucumber, or dilute a small amount of unsweetened cranberry juice into our water. It enhances the flavor, supports liver and kidney detoxification, and even reduces the glycemic index of food.

Should You Use a Water Filter?

Why not drink water that is as close to what Mother Nature intended for us as is possible that doesn't include synthetic chemicals? Filtered water is better for you. It tastes better, too. Another reason to filter your water is that ninety percent of all pharmaceutical drugs ingested are not metabolized and leave the body in urine or feces, ending up in our water supply.

Pharmaceutical drugs and hormones are routinely found in our tap and ground water. This includes psychotropic drugs, hormones from birth control pills, and steroids[42].

It is possible that these extra drugs in the water have to do with the changes found in human and animal hormone levels. You can see it best in amphibians and fish. Their gestation rate is so quick, you can see the effects of substances on many generations that you cannot easily see in mammals or humans. Look at the evidence and then make the decision whether you need to do something for your own health and drink better water.

There are four types of water filtration methods: gravity filters, reverse osmosis, negative ion generators, and distillers. Distilled water removes all minerals as well as chemicals, so unless you are replacing your minerals through supplements, we advise that you drink filtered water, instead.

There is more to the benefits of hydration than just drinking water from filters, though. There is the type of water to consider. Let's look at alkaline and hydrogen-rich water and review their benefits.

Benefits of Alkaline Water

Alkaline water is water with a pH level of more than 7, which is the neutral number between acid and alkaline. So, alkaline water will typically have levels of 8 or 9. It has been promoted for many years as beneficial for the body and many people have experienced those benefits.

We are going to discuss some of the benefits below, but it is important to understand that the stomach is acidic for a reason; it requires acid to digest food. Antiacids are alkaline and neutralize stomach acid, which can impair digestion. Alkaline water also has this ability, so we suggest that you drink it at appropriate times.

So, why is it so popular? There are lots of studies available that show how drinking alkaline water can help with a number of health conditions and even increase longevity in mice. A 3-year study was conducted on 150 mice to see if they lived longer by drinking alkaline water. This study showed that alkaline water provides a higher longevity in terms of 'deceleration aging factor' as compared to the mice that were given regular water[43].

If that isn't enough, it turns out that alkaline water may help reduce the viscosity of blood and help it flow more efficiently. Viscosity is the direct measurement of how efficiently blood flows through the vessels. A study of 100 people found a significant difference in their whole blood viscosity after consuming high-pH water compared to regular water after a strenuous workout. It reduced their blood viscosity by 6.3 percent compared to 3.36 percent with standard purified drinking water. This means blood flowed more efficiently with alkaline water[44].

What Is Hydrogen Water?

While filtered water is crucial and alkaline water is beneficial, you can take your health to a new level by also drinking hydrogen water. This is simply pure water with extra hydrogen molecules added to it. Water molecules consist of two hydrogen atoms and one oxygen atom. It's thought that the body can't effectively absorb the hydrogen in plain water, as it's bound to oxygen. So, when extra hydrogen is added, these hydrogen molecules are "free" and are more accessible to your body.

Now, some alkaline water is hydrogen water, and some is not; it depends on the mineral used to modify the water. It has been shown that both alkaline and electrolyzed water act to suppress free radical levels in living organisms, thereby resulting in disease prevention.

Benefits of Hydrogen Water

Hydrogen water regulates production of our body's own natural antioxidants, such as glutathione and enzymes such as *catalase* and superoxide. Molecular hydrogen is not a direct antioxidant, but rather helps regulate the production of antioxidants and nitric oxide. It even regulates the production of proteins that are either pro- or anti-inflammatory, which can reduce inflammation in the body.

There are numerous amazing studies on hydrogen water. A review named 'A New Approach for the Prevention and Treatment of Cardiovascular Disorders: Molecular Hydrogen Significantly Reduces the Effects of Oxidative Stress'[45] is very useful in explaining in detail how hydrogen, including hydrogen water acts to reduce oxidative stress in cardiovascular disorders. It discusses the damaging impact of oxidative stress on the cells and vessels. You might recall that after an ischemic attack (a restriction in blood supply to tissues) the blood is 're-perfused' into the capillaries, and this is where the glycocalyx is destroyed and needs to rebuild. This is called a 'lethal reperfusion injury.' Hydrogen water has been shown in numerous studies to help the endothelium recover from this injury and, consequently, its glycocalyx.

Hydration Tips

- Caffeinated or alcoholic drinks dehydrate you. You need to drink extra water to compensate.
- Non-caffeinated herbal teas do count as water because they are not caffeinated.
- Your body loses water while you sleep, so drink a glass when you wake up. Drinking water in the morning helps flush out the toxins that have accumulated all night.
- It is better to sip water throughout the day than drink two glasses all at once. Sipping water reduces the stress on the

heart (especially if you have heart disease) and gives your body more time to absorb it.

- Drink more water when you exercise to compensate for fluid loss. This may be self-evident, but I think it is important to take time to bring a bottle of water with you when you leave the house to work out.
- Drink more when you are sick. Even though you don't feel like it, you really need to drink more water to help your body recover from various infections. Your body heats up when you have a fever, which can dehydrate you.

DETOXIFY

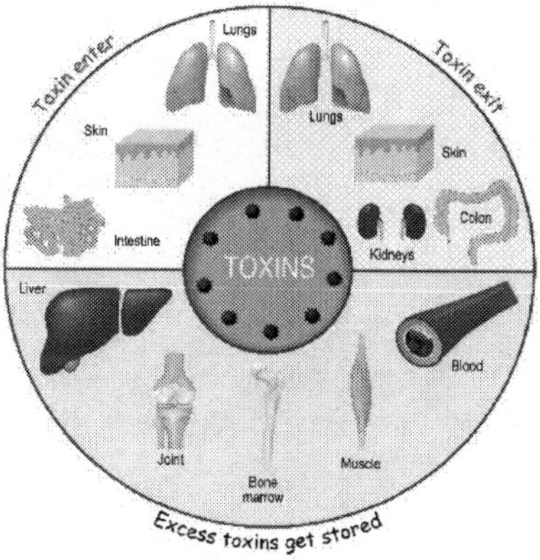

Often people overlook one of the most problematic issues when it comes to maintaining a healthy cardiovascular system—detoxification. Toxins come from industrial processing: refineries, coal burning, power plants, petroleum combustion, nuclear power stations, plastics, textiles, microelectronics, and wood preservation and paper processing plants. These toxins leech into the soil, water, and permeate the air. They are in your food as herbicides and pesticides, in your air as pollutants from carbon monoxide, and other pollutants and even as radiation from the meltdown of nuclear power stations.

You Cannot Escape Toxins

You might not have thought about the effects of toxins on your health and so have not realized how important it is to detoxify. Recent studies have linked exposure to heavy metals, in particular, arsenic, lead, cadmium, and copper to endocrine disruption, which increases the risk of cardiovascular disease, coronary artery disease, diabetes and hypertension according to a review of 37 unique studies[46].

Not to be overlooked, air pollution has been shown to damage endothelial cells! According to a 2006 study, cardiovascular mortality is directly related to pollution. In this longitudinal study of 8111 participants, 1401 died, and 646 of those deaths were due to cardiovascular causes[47].

What causes these pollutants to affect the endothelium? According to the analysis, toxins are deposited in the alveoli from inhaling pollutants. These cause oxidative stress and systemic inflammation, which then causes endothelial dysfunction due to vasoconstriction and hypertension and also cause increased blood viscosity. It is essentially the oxidative stress that adversely impacts the endothelium (and the glycocalyx).

These toxins are everywhere. The entire planet is infected with toxins. Wind, rain, and water carry them, and even if you are living on organic food, you are still being assaulted by toxins!

How to Remove Environmental Toxins and Heavy Metals

If you want to reduce the load placed on your glycocalyx by toxins, then read carefully because you can effectively detoxify heavy metals and toxic compounds from the body. You can use them to create greater balance in your body and improve your well-being by eliminating toxins and pathogens you pick up in the course of living.

We are reviewing four detoxifiers here. You can read through them and pick one or two and notice what happens to your body, in terms of energy, vitality, and immunity.

Activated Charcoal

Activated charcoal is a fine black powder made from bone char, coconut shells, peat, petroleum coke, coal, olive pits, or sawdust. It traps toxins, gas, and chemicals in the body, allowing them to be flushed out so the body doesn't reabsorb them.

The charcoal's porous texture has a negative electrical charge, (You will see this theme throughout this section), which causes it to attract positively charged trap toxins, viruses, and other chemicals in the gut[48]. Because activated charcoal is not absorbed by your body, it can carry the toxins bound to its surface out of your body in feces. It can also help with indigestion and gas.

Bentonite Clay

Bentonite clay, also called *Montmorillonite* clay, is a tasteless detoxifier that works wonders on a bloated gut and for toxicity. It has been used for centuries around the world. Bentonite clay is composed of ash made from volcanos.

The main benefit of bentonite clay is that it draws toxins from the body and provides a range of minerals, including calcium, magnesium, silica, sodium, copper, iron, and potassium. It also benefits the body because it has the ability to produce a type of electric charge when it comes in contact with liquid, so when the clay touches any type of fluid (normally water), it takes on a different charge, which will bind to any toxins that are present in the fluid. When you drink it, it will absorb the toxins and gas, and thereby reduce the inflammation in the gut. By removing toxins, chemicals, and heavy metals in the gut, bentonite clay will promote digestion and even kill viruses.

Diatomaceous Earth

Diatomaceous earth (DE) is a natural product made of fossilized remains of tiny, aquatic organisms called diatoms, whose cell walls are made of biogenic silica. Diatomaceous earth usually comes in the form of a white powder, which is used in water filtering, food manufacturing, skin products and farming. It naturally eliminates free radicals, viruses, insects, parasites, and other harmful organisms by binding to them[49].

When eaten, DE can improve the body's use of calcium, help mineralize bone, and protect joints. The silica within DE helps with normal bone metabolism and joint formation, with evidence over the past 30 years suggesting a positive association between dietary silicon intake and better bone mineral density. Scientists believe it is possible that silicon helps synthesize collagen[50].

FULVIC ACID

Fulvic acid is one of two classes of humic acids, which are organic compounds found in soil, rock sediments, and bodies of water. Over the past several decades, scientists have learned how humic substances found in dirt, including fulvic acid, can actually improve human gut health and, therefore, immune function.

Humic acids are beneficial for digestion and improving energy because of their detoxifying abilities. They are also capable of binding to and breaking down toxins and metals that enter the body. Studies have found that they have ion-selective electrodes that can be used to attract heavy metals, which can significantly improve and detoxify the body.

There is some evidence that fulvic acid's electrolytes can help reduce swelling, decrease inflammation, relax muscles, and improve circulation. Fulvic acid also contains nutrients that improve gut health, including trace minerals, electrolytes, fatty acids, silica, prebiotics, and probiotics. It can also remove waste products from the cells. Fulvic acid can significantly improve the ratio of bacteria living in the gut and help to reduce many digestive symptoms such as constipation, bloating, diarrhea, and food sensitivities.

ZEOLITE

If you are looking for a potent detoxifier, you can also look into Zeolite, as many people swear by it for radiation detoxification. Zeolite is a volcanic mineral which is a porous rock that, when suspended in water, is another silica-based product that has the ability to detoxify the body, similar to DE, bentonite clay, and fulvic acid. It has honeycomb-like structure that contains a negative charge. This negative charge attracts positively charged toxins like lead, mercury, or nitrosamines.[51] Most of the studies done with zeolite used rats or shellfish, so while it is not toxic as a supplement, there is no solid research that it removes toxins in people.

RELAX AND DE-STRESS

As stated earlier, one of the most important inflammation triggers is stress. When stress is out of control, your hormones get out of control and contribute to a damaged glycocalyx. Our bodies are built to manage stress – for short periods of time. Stress reactions are necessary for the fight or flight response when we are put into dangerous or threatening situations.

The problem occurs when stress is chronic and sustained over a long period of time as happens with most people with today's hectic living schedules. The vessels constrict, the glycocalyx becomes damaged and breaks down which inhibits the blood flow over time, then the vessels break down and the cells and tissues are not fed.

- Blood thickens
- Increased blood pressure
- Shallow breathing
- Reduced digestive enzymes
- Tired, foggy, forgetful
- Trembling can occur
- Chills and sweating

Therefore, it is critical that you manage stress to maintain a healthy glycocalyx. To do this, you must put a priority on recreation, relaxation, and rejuvenation. Some people think they are doing something wrong if they take time off. This is not at all the case. Understanding the importance of recharging yourself with downtime is critical to operate at peak performance and avoid the burnout of overwork.

Do something different! Take a walk, play a game, find a quiet place, do yoga, focused breathing, read or even nap. Spend some time with family and friends in a completely loving social environment. Have fun.

And finally, work on getting more sleep. We seem to have a pride in how little we sleep. Sleep is necessary for rejuvenation and those who are not getting enough, increase their odds of obesity, cancer, diabetes, and other health problems associated with an unhealthy glycocalyx.

REFERENCES PART THREE

1. Bruno, R. R., Reed, M., Bimpong-Buta, N. Y., Muessig, J. M., Masyuk, M., Binneboessel, S., Franz, M., Kelm, M., & Jung, C. (2020). Sublingual microcirculation in prehospital critical care medicine: A proof-of-concept study. *Microcirculation (New York, N.Y. : 1994)*, *27*(5), e12614. https://doi.org/10.1111/micc.12614
2. https://glycocheck.com/
3. http://itera.care/
4. Bohn, W., Hess, L., & Burger, R. (2013). The effects of the "physical BEMER® vascular therapy", a method for the physical stimulation of the vasomotion of precapillary microvessels in case of impaired microcirculation, on sleep, pain and quality of life of patients with different clinical pictures on the basis of three scientifically validated scales. Journal of complementary & integrative medicine, 10(Suppl), S5–S13. https://doi.org/10.1515/jcim-2013-0037
5. https://www.avacen.com/
6. https://www.heartfit.ca/external-counterpulsation-therapy-ecp-eecp-calgary-alberta-canada/
7. Fitton, JH. Stringer, DN. Karpiniec, SS. (2015) Review. Therapies from fucoidan: an update. Mar Drugs 13:5920-5946. https://www.ncbi.nlm.nih.gov/pmc/articles/PMC4584361/pdf/marinedrugs-13-05920.pdf
8. Fitton, JH. Brown marine algae: a survey of therapeutic potentials. Alt Comp Therapy 2003; 9:29-33. https://doi.org/10.1089/10762800360520767.
9. Baker, A.B. (2020) Glycocalyx mimetic polysaccharides as therapeutics for atherosclerosis University of Texas Austin, Austin, TX, United States. https://grantome.com/grant/NIH/R21-EB024147-01A1.

10. Zaporozhets, T., & Besednova, N. (2016). Prospects for the therapeutic application of sulfated polysaccharides of brown algae in diseases of the cardiovascular system: review. Pharmaceutical biology, 54(12), 3126–3135. https://doi.org/10.1080/13880209.2016.1185444
11. Reid SNS, Ryu J. K, Kim Y., et al. (2018). The effects of fermented laminaria japonica on short-term working memory and physical fitness in the elderly. Evidence-Based Complementary and Alternative Medicine. https://www.alzdiscovery.org/cognitive-vitality/ratings/fucoidan.
12. Ramachandran, C., Wilk, B., Melnick, S. J., & Eliaz, I. (2017). Synergistic Antioxidant and Anti-Inflammatory Effects between Modified Citrus Pectin and Honokiol. *Evidence-Based Complementary and Alternative Medicine: eCAM,2017*, 8379843. https://doi.org/10.1155/2017/8379843
13. Eliaz, I., Weil, E., & Wilk, B. (2007). Integrative medicine and the role of modified citrus pectin/alginates in heavy metal chelation and detoxification--five case reports. *Forschende Komplementarmedizin (2006), 14*(6), 358–364. https://doi.org/10.1159/000109829
14. Li, Z. H., Gao, X., Chung, V. C., Zhong, W. F., Fu, Q., Lv, Y. B., Wang, et al. (2020). Associations of regular glucosamine use with all-cause and cause-specific mortality: a large prospective cohort study. Annals of the rheumatic diseases, 79(6), 829–836. https://doi.org/10.1136/annrheumdis-2020-217176
15. Al'Qteishat, A., Gaffney, J., Krupinski, J., Rubio, F., West, D., Kumar, S., Kumar, P., Mitsios, N., & Slevin, M. (2006). Changes in hyaluronan production and metabolism following ischaemic stroke in man. Brain: a journal of neurology, 129(Pt 8), 2158–2176. https://doi.org/10.1093/brain/awl139

16. Bałan, B. J., Niemcewicz, M., Kocik, J., Jung, L., Skopińska-Różewska, E., & Skopiński, P. (2014). Oral administration of Aloe vera gel, anti-microbial and anti-inflammatory herbal remedy, stimulates cell-mediated immunity and antibody production in a mouse model. *Central-European journal of immunology*, *39*(2), 125–130. https://doi.org/10.5114/ceji.2014.43711
17. Rienks, J., Barbaresko, J., & Nöthlings, U. (2017). Association of Polyphenol Biomarkers with Cardiovascular Disease and Mortality Risk: A Systematic Review and Meta-Analysis of Observational Studies. *Nutrients*, *9*(4), 415. https://doi.org/10.3390/nu9040415
18. Lockyer, S., Rowland, I., Spencer, J.P.E. *et al.* Impact of phenolic-rich olive leaf extract on blood pressure, plasma lipids and inflammatory markers: a randomised controlled trial. *Eur J Nutr* 56, 1421–1432 (2017). https://doi.org/10.1007/s00394-016-1188-y
19. Vogel, P., Kasper Machado, I., Garavaglia, J., Zani, V. T., de Souza, D., & Morelo Dal Bosco, S. (2014). Polyphenols benefits of olive leaf (Olea europaea L) to human health. Nutricion hospitalaria, 31(3), 1427–1433. https://doi.org/10.3305/nh.2015.31.3.8400
20. Olmez, E., Vural, K., Gok, S., Ozturk, Z., Kayalar, H., Ayhan, S., & Var, A. (2015). Olive Leaf Extract Improves the Atherogenic Lipid Profile in Rats Fed a High Cholesterol Diet. Phytotherapy research: PTR, 29(10), 1652–1657. https://doi.org/10.1002/ptr.5445
21. Cortés Castell, E., Veciana Galindo, C., Torro Montell, L., Sirvent Segura, E., Rizo Baeza, M. M., & Gil Guillén, V. (2014). Actividad antiinflamatoria de un extracto polifenólico de hueso de olivas en la línea celular de monocitos humanos THP1-XBLUE-CD14 [Anti-inflammatory activity of olive seed polyphenolic extract in the THP1-XBLUE-CD14 human monocytes cell line].

Nutricion hospitalaria, 30(1), 113–117. https://doi.org/10.3305/nh.2014.30.1.7482

22. Breuss, J. M., Atanasov, A. G., & Uhrin, P. (2019). Resveratrol and Its Effects on the Vascular System. International journal of molecular sciences, 20(7), 1523. https://doi.org/10.3390/ijms20071523
23. Cutler, B. R., Gholami, S., Chua, J. S., Kuberan, B., & Anandh Babu, P. V. (2018). Blueberry metabolites restore cell surface glycosaminoglycans and attenuate endothelial inflammation in diabetic human aortic endothelial cells. *International journal of cardiology, 261,* 155–158. https://doi.org/10.1016/j.ijcard.2018.03.027
24. Patade, A., Devareddy, L., Lucas, E. A., Korlagunta, K., Daggy, B. P., & Arjmandi, B. H. (2008). Flaxseed reduces total and LDL cholesterol concentrations in Native American postmenopausal women. *Journal of women's health (2002), 17*(3), 355–366. https://doi.org/10.1089/jwh.2007.0359
25. Adolphe, J. L., Whiting, S. J., Juurlink, B. H., Thorpe, L. U., & Alcorn, J. (2010). Health effects with consumption of the flax lignan secoisolariciresinol diglucoside. *The British journal of nutrition, 103*(7), 929–938. https://doi.org/10.1017/S0007114509992753
26. Sharma, S. K., Vij, A. S., & Sharma, M. (2013). Mechanisms and clinical uses of capsaicin. *European journal of pharmacology. 720*(1-3), 55–62. https://doi.org/10.1016/j.ejphar.2013.10.053
27. Chopan, M., & Littenberg, B. (2017). The Association of Hot Red Chili Pepper Consumption and Mortality: A Large Population-Based Cohort Study. *PloS one, 12*(1), e0169876. https://doi.org/10.1371/journal.pone.0169876

28. Bonaccio, M., Di Castelnuovo, A., Costanzo, S., Ruggiero, E., De Curtis, A., Persichillo, M., Tabolacci, C., Facchiano, F., Cerletti, C., Donati, M. B., de Gaetano, G., Iacoviello, L., & Moli-sani Study Investigators (2019). Chili Pepper Consumption and Mortality in Italian Adults. *Journal of the American College of Cardiology, 74*(25), 3139–3149. https://doi.org/10.1016/j.jacc.2019.09.068
29. Barbul A. (1986). Arginine: biochemistry, physiology, and therapeutic implications. *JPEN. Journal of parenteral and enteral nutrition, 10*(2), 227–238. https://doi.org/10.1177/0148607186010002227
30. Allerton, T. D., Proctor, D. N., Stephens, J. M., Dugas, T. R., Spielmann, G., & Irving, B. A. (2018). l-Citrulline Supplementation: Impact on Cardiometabolic Health. *Nutrients, 10*(7), 921. https://doi.org/10.3390/nu10070921
31. Salem, M.B., Affes, H., Ksouda, K. *et al.* Pharmacological Studies of Artichoke Leaf Extract and Their Health Benefits. *Plant Foods Hum Nutr* 70, 441–453 (2015). https://doi.org/10.1007/s11130-015-0503-8
32. Ahmed, S. F., Abd Al Haleem, E. N., & El-Tantawy, W. H. (2019). Evaluation of the anti-atherogenic potential of Egyptian artichoke leaf extract in hypercholesterolemic rats. *Archives of physiology and biochemistry*, 1–12. Advance online publication. https://doi.org/10.1080/13813455.2019.1669662
33. Schwalfenberg, G. K. (2017). Vitamins K1 and K2: The Emerging Group of Vitamins Required for Human Health. *Journal of nutrition and metabolism, 2017*, 6254836. https://doi.org/10.1155/2017/6254836
34. Kidd P. M. (2010). Vitamins D and K as pleiotropic nutrients: clinical importance to the skeletal and cardiovascular systems and preliminary evidence for

synergy. *Alternative medicine review: a journal of clinical therapeutic, 15*(3), 199–222. https://pubmed.ncbi.nlm.nih.gov/21155624/

35. Goldberg, R. J., & Katz, J. (2007). A meta-analysis of the analgesic effects of omega-3 polyunsaturated fatty acid supplementation for inflammatory joint pain. *Pain, 129*(1-2), 210–223. https://doi.org/10.1016/j.pain.2007.01.020
36. Chau, J. Y., Grunseit, A. C., Chey, T., Stamatakis, E., Brown, W. J., Matthews, C. E., Bauman, A. E., & van der Ploeg, H. P. (2013). Daily sitting time and all-cause mortality: a meta-analysis. *PloS one, 8*(11), e80000. https://doi.org/10.1371/journal.pone.0080000
37. Rachel Ballard-Barbash, Christine M. Friedenreich, Kerry S. Courneya, Sameer M. Siddiqi, Anne McTiernan, Catherine M. Alfano, Physical Activity, Biomarkers, and Disease Outcomes in Cancer Survivors: A Systematic Review, *JNCI: Journal of the National Cancer Institute*, Volume 104, Issue 11, 6 June 2012, Pages 815–840, https://doi.org/10.1093/jnci/djs207
38. Schmitz, B., Niehues, H., Lenders, M., Thorwesten, L., Klose, A., Krüger, M., Brand, E., & Brand, S. M. (2019). Effects of high-intensity interval training on microvascular glycocalyx and associated microRNAs. American journal of physiology. Heart and circulatory physiology, 316(6), H1538–H1551. https://doi.org/10.1152/ajpheart.00751.2018
39. Vital capacity as a predictor of cardiovascular disease: (1983). The Framingham Study. American Heart Journal. Volume 105, Issue 2, February 1983, Pages 311-315. https://www.sciencedirect.com/sdfe/pdf/download/eid/1-s2.0-000287038390532X/first-page-pdf.
40. Goodman, A. B., Blanck, H. M., Sherry, B., Park, S., Nebeling, L., & Yaroch, A. L. (2013). Behaviors and attitudes associated with low drinking water intake among US adults, Food Attitudes and Behaviors Survey,

2007. Preventing chronic disease, 10, E51.
https://doi.org/10.5888/pcd10.120248

41. Hahn R. G. (2020). Water content of the endothelial glycocalyx layer estimated by volume kinetic analysis. *Intensive care medicine experimental, 8*(1), 29. https://doi.org/10.1186/s40635-020-00317-z
42. Bexfield, L.M., Toccalino, P.L., Belitz, K., Foreman, W.T., and Furlong, E.T. (2019) Hormones and Pharmaceuticals in Groundwater Used As a Source of Drinking Water Across the United States. Environmental Science & Technology 53(6), 2950-2960. https://DOI.org/10.1021/acs.est.8b05592
43. Magro, M., Corain, L., Ferro, S., Baratella, D., Bonaiuto, E., Terzo, M., Corraducci, V., Salmaso, L., & Vianello, F. (2016). Alkaline Water and Longevity: A Murine Study. Evidence-based complementary and alternative medicine: eCAM, 2016, 3084126. https://doi.org/10.1155/2016/3084126
44. Weidman, J., Holsworth, R. E., Jr, Brossman, B., Cho, D. J., St Cyr, J., & Fridman, G. (2016). Effect of electrolyzed high-pH alkaline water on blood viscosity in healthy adults. Journal of the International Society of Sports Nutrition, 13, 45. https://doi.org/10.1186/s12970-016-0153-8
45. LeBaron, T. W., Kura, B., Kalocayova, B., Tribulova, N., & Slezak, J. (2019). A New Approach for the Prevention and Treatment of Cardiovascular Disorders. Molecular Hydrogen Significantly Reduces the Effects of Oxidative Stress. Molecules (Basel, Switzerland), 24(11), 2076. https://doi.org/10.3390/molecules24112076
46. Yang, A. M., Lo, K., Zheng, T. Z., Yang, J. L., Bai, Y. N., Feng, Y. Q., Cheng, N., & Liu, S. M. (2020). Environmental heavy metals and cardiovascular diseases: Status and future direction. *Chronic diseases and translational medicine*, *6*(4), 251–259. https://doi.org/10.1016/j.cdtm.2020.02.005
47. Nodari, S., Corulli, A., Manerba, A., Metra, M., Apostoli, P., & Dei Cas, L. (2006). Endothelial damage due to air

pollution. Heart international, 2(2), 115. https://doi.org/10.4081/hi.2006.115

48. Clark, K. J., Sarr, A. B., Grant, P. G., Phillips, T. D., & Woode, G. N. (1998). In vitro studies on the use of clay, clay minerals and charcoal to adsorb bovine rotavirus and bovine coronavirus. Veterinary microbiology, 63(2-4), 137–146. https://doi.org/10.1016/s0378-1135(98)00241-7.
49. Introduction to Bacillariophyta (The Diatoms). UC Berkeley. https://ucmp.berkeley.edu/chromista/bacillariophyta.html.
50. Diatoms. *Wikipedia*. https://en.wikipedia.org/wiki/Diatom
51. Topashka-Ancheva, M., Beltcheva, M., Metcheva, R., Rojas, J. A., Rodriguez-De la Fuente, A. O., Gerasimova, T., Rodríguez-Flores, L. E., & Teodorova, S. E. (2012). Modified natural clinoptilolite detoxifies small mammal's organism loaded with lead II: genetic, cell, and physiological effects. *Biological trace element research, 147*(1-3), 206–216. https://doi.org/10.1007/s12011-011-9289-1

CONCLUSION

At the risk of being too redundant, we would like to make one more analogy to drive home why this information is so important. You probably have a circuit breaker or fuse box in your home that is designed to protect your home's entire electrical system. It does this by breaking before you have an incident that would cause major electrical damage or fire in your home. In a way, your capillaries are similar to this. They break down before you get to the point of a heart attack or stroke. This gives you a chance to repair and prevent further damage before it's too late. We now have technology that can detect this early breakdown so that you can do something about it!

It is our hope that you will have taken this information and absorbed it so that, no matter your age or state of health, you can now become actively involved in improving your microvascular circulation for better health and longevity.

Other Health Books by Carol Merlo, M.Ed.

No Achy Joints

Discoveries on the Path to a Pain Free Body

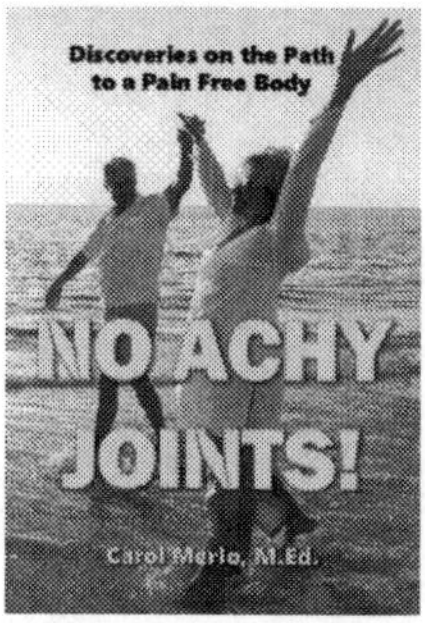

No Achy Joints shares the journey that so many people who are dealing with arthritis take and who end up spending thousands of dollars on pills and practitioners, only to get worse.

Carol Merlo, M.Ed., has walked that same path and has found methods that actually work. This book will help you wade through the confusing mountains of hype and give you a clear path to having a pain free body. In this book, you will learn:

- The Role of Inflammation in Joint Pain
- Supplements that Really Work
- Foods That Make a Difference
- How Hormone Imbalances Cause Joint Pain
- Why You Have to Move
- What to Do If it Still Hurts

Create a Happy Body

The 8 Golden Keys to a Lifetime of Wellness

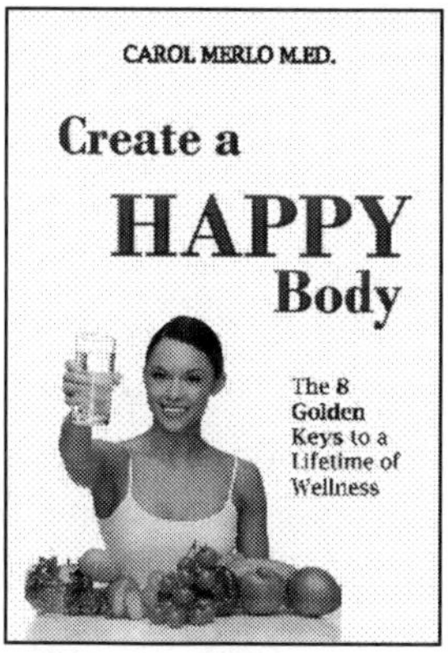

Do you want great health and wellness but are confused by all the information coming at you?

What if you could tap into simple and effective tools to maintain health and wellness and experience greater happiness and vitality? If you don't feel "quite right" then it's time to Create a Happy Body. Find out how easy it is to make a couple of simple shifts to transform your energy and pain levels. Whether you want insights into greater mental health or strategies for improving your longevity, you will find your answers here.

There are numerous pills, diet drinks, and healthy living techniques that promise a "healthy you." Despite that, many still find health and wellness out of reach.

But what if there were a simple path you could take to bring about the well-being that we all desire? In Create a

Happy Body, you'll discover that it is possible to feel good, stay motivated, avoid the doctor, and more by following the 8 steps to a healthy mind and body.

Discover. . .

- **How to stick to your goals** to get leaner and feel better
- How to overcome the single biggest obstacle to creating the life you want
- How our food supply became toxic and **what you can do to protect yourself**
- A simple guideline that will drastically improve how you eat
- What **Superfoods** can do to transform your health
- How you can **have fun** getting the exercise you need
- The most important thing you can do to extend your life --- and it's FREE!
- How to overcome emotional ups and downs that create stress and negatively impact your happiness.

Now you can Look & Feel More Healthy, Youthful, Vibrant, & Beautiful!

Don't wait! The aging clock is ticking. Only you can take charge to prevent the ravages of a toxic, nutrient deprived environment from taking its toll on your body. Buy Create a Happy Body today!

The Hemp Miracle:

How One Miraculous Plant Is Healing the Planet and Its People

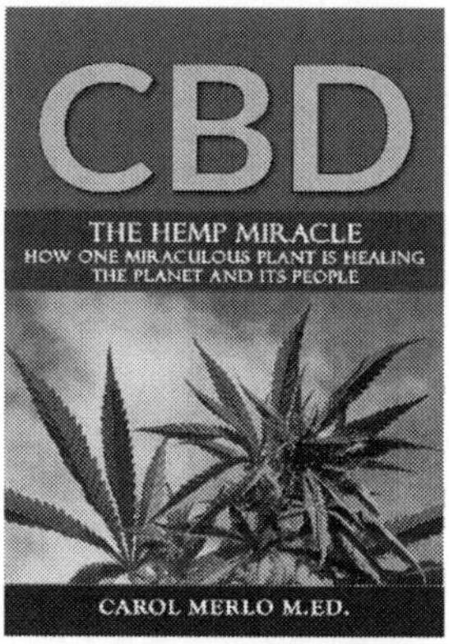

This practical guide to understanding CBD and industrial hemp products is a detailed, yet easy-to-read tool for anyone who wants to feel better without wading through the fluff and buy products that work. Take it from someone who knows what it is like to be in pain and hates the hype.

In this Book You'll Discover:

- Why you need CBD
- An overview of the endocannabinoid system
- How CBD is made
- The research that has been done on health conditions
- How to buy safe, quality products
- How much to take
- The fascinating history of hemp throughout the ages
- The science behind CBD's health benefits, both as a food and as a dietary supplement.
- The many industrial uses of hemp, including green housing, fuel, and plastics

- **The legal status of hemp and CBD across the world.**

You don't need to suffer from nagging pains and anxiety. Read this book and change your life!

Made in the USA
Monee, IL
20 August 2024

64218072R00090